Gastric Band Hypnosis for Rapid Weight Loss

Reprogram Your Brain and Lose Weight in Less
than 10 Days. Stop Emotional Eating and Heal Yourself.
The Natural Non-Invasive
Technique to Feel Less Hungry

David Baxter

DISCLAIMER NOTICE

III

INTRODUCTION

For people seeking relief from their weight loss issues, you'll find this guide a perfect resource to equip you with the right knowledge on the basics of Hypno-Band with effective techniques to stop food addiction with quick and permanent weight loss, meditation, eat healthy food, and emotional eating suppression.

People had hesitated about hypnosis in the earlier times because of the thought that it contains evil forces or anything that suggests negativity. It's been related to influencing someone to commit corruption of any kind. Because of this, people are excited to try it out. However, what they did not know is that there are a variety of advantages that can be obtained from this approach when performed correctly and with the aid of the right people.

What Hypnosis Can Treat It can stimulate the functions of a person's body and, among others, can relieve someone from common sleep and digestive disorders. It can build some harmony in one's personality and approach to life, too. For one thing, the right hypnotic therapy will put away one of the things that hinder you from optimizing your procrastination ability.

Hypnosis operates by making the human subconscious focus on something unforgettable or pleasant to provide the body with rhythm. The body may also adjust to a pattern until it usually continues on its own. It's also even more shocking to remember that hypnosis is also an effective weight loss option. But how does one really do it?

Starting out with hypnosis, there are guidelines for hypnosis, which could be very helpful. For starters, of course, all the requisite training that correlates with the approach will have to be taken. It should be remembered that while hypnosis offers a person many benefits, it can also pose dangers when performed in the wrong way and without proper planning. Gathering all possible hypnosis tips from different sources wouldn't hurt one.

There are now several books available and write-ups on the subject as well as the site online about the process, so this one should be simple. However, the safest approach is for the experts themselves to demonstrate. An individual may already proceed to actually perform hypnotism when all of this is finished. The first important thing to concentrate one's attention is to evaluate the subject carefully. Anything that annoys an individual needs to be exposed or found. This will serve as the basis for the subsequent acts. For a hypnotic therapist, what you want for your patient is to unload everything first and start with a clear mind if you are doing it for yourself.

Hypnotherapy helps someone who is willing to learn and is ready to fix aspects of their lives that they are dissatisfied with. Simply, it heals into an altered state of consciousness. Experienced experiences are analogous to reaching deep relaxation, and the therapist accesses the subconscious mind where important changes for emotional and physiological problems can be made. To gain even more from hypnotherapy, it helps if the client has faith and trust in the therapist and so it is crucial for the client to ensure that all specific questions are addressed before beginning the sessions, and that will start the treatment correctly.

CHAPTER 1

WHAT IS A GASTRIC BAND?

It fills up quickly and slows your consumption rate. The band shows you whenever you make healthy food options, reduce appetite, and limit food intake and volume. However, it leaves you with a problematic bariatric surgery option, which is a drastic step that carries risks and pains like any other gastrointestinal surgical operation.

Hypnotic Gastric Band

The hypnotic gastric band is the natural healthy eating tool that will help control your appetite and portion sizes. In this sense, hypnosis plays a significant role in helping you to lose weight without having to go through the risk that comes with surgery. It is a subconscious suggestion that you already have, a gastric band comes in- tending to influence the body to respond by creating a feeling of satiety. It is now available in the public domain that dieting does not help solve weight loss and management's lifestyle challenges. Temporary diet plans are not practical while maintaining continuous programs is complicated. Notably, these plans are going to deprive you of your favorite foods since they're too restrictive. Deep down within you, you might have a problem with your body's weight since diets have not worked for you in the past.

You must try hypnosis by reaching this point, which has proven some results in aiding weight loss.

Does it really work?

Usually, the conscious mind is receptive to suggestions because it usually analyzes it. With hypnosis, you will reach your desired weight, become healthier, and stay in shape for life with the right mindset. This way, you will be able to reframe your thinking patterns because of all the tips and disassociation principles. With the hypnotic gastric band, you will use ecommendations to influence a different response from your body triggered by sensory data to create a new reality. The suggestions will be to provide a guideline for you to follow without questioning or critiquing. Ultimately, this power will allow you to reframe and reshape your perception regarding a specific behavior. The complex network in your brain has many different interpretations of the world around you, and the most unhelpful and negative thoughts have worked their way into that network. Thus, you become susceptible to uncontrolled unconscious urges, likening and ignoring bodyweight concerns. Hypnotic gastric band will help you to be able to dampen and overcome all those wild thoughts, believes, and suggestions that are allowing you to alter your behavior.

Powerful Affirmations

You should change your lifestyle if you want to have experience permanent weight loss or control. Powerful affirmations are essential in helping to change your life- style slowly. Thus, you should practice regular affirmations for weight loss to realize your dream of losing weight. Notably, weight control is a direct function of your lifestyle because you are solely responsible for your behavior. You can use effective weight loss affirmations to be able to initiate these measures from your mind. Thus, you should change your thinking; otherwise, no form of dieting will ever help. Weight loss affirmations are significant in your mind, as they allow you to become a comfort in your desired weight. You should also consider your affirmations' words to ensure that you focus on the solution and not the problem. For instance, you shouldn't say "I am not that fat" because that is the problem that you're saying.

You are repeatedly repeating these words, which will help show that you are determined to take the bold step of living and fitter life.

Therefore, here are the words:

I weigh _____ pounds: this affirmation states the desired weight in your mind instantly, and as you repeat the words, you are reminding yourself about your destiny and all measures that you should take. I will achieve my ideal weight to enhance my physical fitness: you are embracing a lighter weight and improving your physical activity. I love eating healthy food because they help me to be able to attain my ideal weight: This statement promotes healthy eating and cravings for healthy food. I ease digestion by chewing all my food to reach my ideal weight: This affirmation is perfect to say before every meal because it guides the rate and amount of food you consume. I am controlling my weight by combining healthy eating, and it helps me to be able to control my appetite and my portion sizes: It is great to repeat this particular affirmation with others in front of a mirror to keep reminding your subconscious mind about your goals. Also, these affirmations work best when you're meditating or in a trance state. The combination will help to do wonders in your weight loss endeavor.

Powerful Visualization

With the hypnotic gastric band, you can use your imagination to control your subconscious mind and your body. Visualizing weight loss means that you're creating the image of how you want to be in your mind. Visualization is a beautiful tool that triggers your subconscious mind so that you can shape your body to match your mental image. If you visualize according to the way you're supposed to imagine, you will lose weight, improve your looks, and become more energetic. You have to realize that your emotions and thoughts affect your body, either for better or worse. Negative thinking, fear, anger, worry, and stress, harm the body, which then produces toxins that will drastically affect you. Now, if you are happy, positive, and confident, you will be able to energize and strengthen your body. Learning how to use your subconscious mind during visualization is for your advantage. It is a mental diet, which you need to incorporate into your weight loss plan. Visualization is an excellent thing because it helps you to overcome overeating and emotional eating. The significance of visualization is not in your physical body but in the feelings of overcoming your obsessions and challenges with your food, weight, perfect body, plagues, and the restrictions that are keeping you on a diet merry go round. With this hypnotic gastric band, you will realize that visualization is a simple process, and it dramatically helps during weight loss. Find some frequent moments where you will be able to sit down for several minutes and visualize your slim body. Ignore all the doubts, worries, and negative thoughts and just focus on the image. Forget your current looks and imagine such a beautiful, slim, and ideal weight. Imagine how gorgeous you look in your swimming suit and the tight clothing you always want to wear. Visualize how your peers and your family are complimenting your slim body and slim looks. Watch the entire scene as if it is real and happening right in front of you. Feel free to construct the different versions of these instances or your other physical roles like dancing or swimming. Visualize the compliments that you're hearing from people about your slim body, and watch them those people as they admiringly glare at you.

Ensure that the images you create in your mind are colorful, realistic, and real. See yourself in each of these natural and exciting scenes with your ideal weight. Avoid using words that might destroy all the efforts that you've put into and allow only the thoughts of your ideal weight and shape to come to your mind. Powerful visualizations will work wonders when you practice hypnosis because it makes the mental image a possible reality.

Just watch the whole scene as if it is real and happening now.

- Feel free to construct different versions of these instances or other physical roles, such as dancing or swimming. Visualize yourself hearing compliments from other people about your slim body and watch them admiringly glare at you.

- Make the images you make in your mind colorful, realistic, and alive. See yourself in each of these real and exciting scenes in the ideal weight.

Avoid words that may destroy the efforts you may have made and let only the thoughts of your ideal weight and shape into your mind. Powerful visualization works wonders when practiced in hypnosis, for it makes the mental image a possible reality.

HOW IT FUNCTIONS

If you would like to lose weight without starvation or yoyo dieting, then the hypnotic gastric band is the ultimate resort. This gastric band does not require surgery but only meditation and hypnosis. Therefore, it offers numerous benefits that make it the solution to rapid weight loss and craving healthy food.

It is pain-free

As opposed to the physical gastric band, the hypnotic gastric band does not require surgery associated with pain and routine follow-ups. Therefore, you don't have to worry about the risks you need to take, as no physical operation will be done on your body. You only need to hypnotize and utilize the hypnosis to work on your body weight.

100% safe

As hypnosis is a non-invasive, non-surgical and safe technique, so is the hypnotic gastric band whose mechanism is initiated in your subconscious mind. Through the practice, there are no expected dangers, and you learn about self-awareness and the course of your life. Time-efficient You do not need to wait for your vacation to acquire a hypnotic gastric band. The tool does not affect your schedule as hypnosis can be combined with most of your day to day activities. You do not need time off to adjust the band or report complications.

No meal replacement or dieting

With the hypnotic gastric band, you do not need to stop eating your most enjoyable food. Instead, you develop a principle that makes you feel in control and enable you to lose weight consistently and naturally without dieting. You exercise and unlock the power in you to make positive changes in life. No complications

No surgery is performed in hypnotic gastric surgery puts away the worry about future complications. The ease in your mind plays a significant role in focusing your mind on the things that matter, such as visualization and meditation. This way, you can put off negative thinking and live your life fearlessly and positively. Helps discover your hidden potential

The use of hypnosis and meditation makes you learn how to use your mind's power to change your perception and erase negative thoughts. Similarly, you become capable of helping not only with weight loss but also with other psychological and social aspects such as confidence. Hypnosis helps plant a subconscious suggestion in your mind making it stick and become a strong idea. Cost-Effective

The hypnotic gastric band does not snatch away your working time, making you fully productive at your workplace with no deductions. In a same way, there are no costs in hypnosis and meditation than the physical gastric band. Positively living your life adds to your savings.

CHAPTER 2

GASTRIC BAND FOR RAPID WEIGHT LOSS

Obesity is rising rapidly globally and is becoming one of the most significant problems for the urban population. Individuals do all kinds of things, mainly physical workouts, to lose weight, but only a small portion takes nutritious foods into ac- count. Over time most people are used to these patterns, making the fight much harder to lose weight. Here weight loss with hypnosis is beneficial, but conclusive findings do not confirm scientifically. Hypnosis's weight loss is not immediate but happens after changing his / her ideas and habits. Therefore, a person begins to lose weight. Hypnotherapists mix images, thoughts, and words and bring them to a person's mind to change the body's picture, perception, and belief. A person prepares to adopt healthy habits to lose weight. Hypnosis can only use to lose weight if done together with other strategies, such as exercise. To be open to this process, you must prepare to hypnotize. Secondly, you need to have complete faith in the hypnotherapist and the techniques used. If you are unable to submit your mind to the guidance of hypnotherapists, it may be a waste of time to undertake the procedure. Besides hypnosis, binaural and isochronic beats use to help them lose weight. These beats help re-program the subconscious mind with frequencies of 4-8 Hz that activate the Theta state of mind.   This state corresponds to a profound trance and easily achieves by skilled mediators. Monaural beats are also instrumental in weight loss, but most people say isochronic tones are much more useful. Such brainwave training mainly influences a person's general health over their weight to alter their minds. By changing the emphasis from weight loss to well-being, the approach begins to change one to a better mental status that benefits from the fact that it attracts the like. Hypnosis, also known as hypnotherapy, refers to the profoundly relaxed, al- most transitory state of people. However, people are far more open to suggestions in this society. When an individual hypnotizes, he is exceptionally calm. You can focus more quickly than "wake up" and consider constructive ideas that enter the subconscious mind. Such suggestions are useful if the person is awake. A strong therapist takes the patient time. They're going to communicate with them. And the therapist can try to communicate with the client in the subconscious while the client becomes hypnotized. The psychiatrist would be just like an investigator who tries to find the underlying factor that triggers abuse or unethical behavior.

Using binaural beats, which clinically prove to work for everyone, one should concentrate on positive body health aspects. As a result, you gain better health and ultimately meet other healthier bodies. The use of binaural weight loss beats is much simpler and faster than different approaches, such as food plans and weight loss pills. Of course, other things need to do so, but binaural beats make the procedure much simpler and more pleasant than weight loss in hypnosis.

Why You Can't Lose weight

People become emotionally attached to food from infancy through adulthood. Children sometimes get rewarded with snacks or treats for healthy behavior; adults can treat to dinner. There are many celebrations across the year, from Christmas, Halloween, Thanksgiving, birthdays, and Valentine's Day. All these celebrations are food-focused, and as people eat together, they feel good and happy. It has also proved that an aroma of a special kind of baked cake can create an emotional connection memory that will last throughout someone's lifetime. Some foods are for nourishment, but others take just for comfort, depending on how they make us feel. Whenever the brain reacts and feels pleasure for a particular food within our reach, we will most of the time grab it and eat it. High body mass index (BMI) link to emotional problems like anxiety, depression, and stress. Those personal issues can make one overindulge after a rough day at the office to reward a good feeling. Some people use junks as a coping mechanism when they hear bad news. This habit can only improve by using meditation exercises to deal with emotions, stress, or anxiety. As the practices continue and you pay close attention to your breath and allocate more time for thinking.

Types of Eating

We eat to survive, and without food, we will die. Our body needs nutrients to function effectively. Eating because one is hungry is different from eating because there is food or food. We need to train our system so that we eat to curb hunger just the same way we drink water to quench thirst. While food lovers explore different kinds of food, most are keen enough to incorporate healthy eating.

Mindful Eating

It is a framework used to bring back one's relationship with food and eating experiences. In this technique, your presence is vital, and all the senses are engaged. For instance, how the food smells, the taste of the food, how delicious it looks, and lastly, your body's reaction to the food. By this, I mean how that particular food made you feel. Mindful eating always incorporates intuitive eating. It makes the body relax and slow down slightly as we listen to inner cues of real hunger. Thus, helping us rectify and reduce emotional binge or emotional eating. Mindful eating can lead to weight loss as long as one makes the right food choices. It is a psychologically controlled type, and the food portion is measured depending on the need. In mind eating, it doesn't matter how much food is there.

What matters is the quantity needed at that particular time. Eating thus becomes a response to hunger other than a leisure activity. People who follow this eating method suffer from obesity. They are physically fit and healthy. During eating also there is no rush regardless of whether one is late or not. The chewing is simultaneous and swallowing.

Intuitive Eating

It is a non-diet approach, mind, and body approach to wellness and health. This approach does not encourage dieting but emphasizes listening to the inner body and hunger cues. By trusting our bodies, intuitive healing renews our relationship with food. Though it does not encourage dieting, it uses nutritional information to make healthy eating choices and habits. By this habit, we eat because we need not because we have to, and dietary values accept without bias. In this method, we rely more on our intuition. Food uses to satisfy a need. Without the inner cue of hunger, no need for food. Those who want to escape dieting stress can appreciate this approach since it is useful and practical. There is no connection between emotions and food in this type of eating.

Emotional or Stress Eating

It happens when people start overeating or under food when overwhelmed with mixed emotions rather than eating in response to their inner cues. Strong emotions we experience can sometimes prevent us from listening to our physical feelings, thus preventing us from feeling hungry or full. In such a scenario, food is used as a coping mechanism, reducing the intense emotion temporarily. This habit is very addictive, and if not controlled, can lead to obesity, rapid weight gain, overeating, guilt, and shame. A stress-related eating dis- order cannot make one vulnerable and not comfortable with the body. Meditation plays a significant role because one will handle stress and, there- fore, not use food as a coping mechanism. Stress eating affects millions of people each year, and although not many will admit it can cause food addiction and unhealthy eating choices. They believe eating relieve them of stress and often blame other people for their problems as one eats. They do not see the need to eat healthy because their mind is preoccupied with so many things.

Dieting

A psychologically controlled type, and the food portion is measured depending on the need. In mind eating, it doesn't matter how much food is there.

What matters is the quantity needed at that particular time. Eating thus becomes a response to hunger other than a leisure activity. People who follow this eating method suffer from obesity. They are physically fit and healthy. During eating also there is no rush regardless of whether one is late or not. The chewing is simultaneous and swallowing.

CHAPTER 3

TACKLING BARRIERS TO WEIGHT LOSS

There are plenty of barriers to weight loss from an individual, to medical, to support mental health and system. Meditation, if incorporated, will bring healthy and fruitful results. Commitment to overcome the challenges as well as to be centered on reaching your goals is significant. There are plenty of distractions, especially before you start a tour weight loss regime.

It will take resilience and discipline to manage a healthy loss program. We have to give weight loss the priority it deserves. Additionally, we have to understand the presence of the said barriers and their contribution toward ours. The walls are going to determine our failures and successes.

Set Goals That Are Realistic

When you set goals, ensure they are attainable, specific, and practical. It is effort- less to work on goals that are realistic and reach them for far better results. How- ever, if the plans are unrealistic, the success rate will be low since one will be discouraged. For instance, when starting with meditation, you'll start with as little as five minutes 1 day and gradually increase it every day until you reach the maximum time of sixty minutes. The same is true for slim down during the meditation process. You can start focusing on losing a few pounds each week and gradually increase until you reach your goal. Nevertheless, as you set goals, realize it is not your fault if they do not work out as you would plan, do your best, and keep your focus.

Always be accountable

When you've decided to commit in meditation to weight loss, don't be shy away from sharing your plan with the support system of yours and family. It's to make sure that the folks you talk about reinforce the commitment and form part of the support system. The way they are going to feel a part of the system and give support whenever there's a need. You can also use apps for timings and reminders; this way, you have a backup plan when you forget. You can also make use of motivational bands when you accomplish a mile- stone set. Being accountable makes you like your successes, acknowledges your failure, and appreciate your support system. People thrive when they feel accountable for something, especially on food advantageous to their well-being.

Modify the mindset of yours

Your thinking must be modified to be keen on the info you're telling yourself.

Ensure your brain does not fill with negative and unproductive thoughts that will bring you down or perhaps discourage you. Don't be scared of challenging the ideas of yours and appreciate the body image of yours. Your mindset determines your thinking and, in turn, creates a feeling of rejection or perhaps appreciation. Our weight loss largely depends on the mood of ours. Do you think you can do it? If you believe you've all it takes, then absolutely nothing will prevent or even stop you.

Manage stress regularly

Having a stress management technique should be part of one's daily routine. You need to develop a healthy stress-relieving mechanism that can help you live a stress-free life. Understand that meditation is a stress reliever in its own right as it helps calm the mind and soothes the body. It can use to manage stress and its benefits fully utilized to live a more productive life. Be able to handle stress efficiently. Focus is not healthy for the mind. If not handle, it can cause emotional problems and makes one irrational, moody, or violent. Be your boss when managing your stress.

Be educated about weight loss

As you embark on meditation for weight loss, be educated about how it works; that way, weight loss will not be a struggle. You will be able to handle failed attempts as well as appreciate the progress made. You will know what you have been doing wrong and decide on the best meditation exercise for you. If you have misleading information, then your general progress may inhibit Weight loss needs to be expensive; neither does it require a costly gym membership or enrollment in a costly meditation class. There are various self-practice meditation exercises that you can comfortably do at home. Different meal plans and diets may work for others though they may not offer long-term solutions or lasting behavior changes. Have the right information that you need. Don't be misled by anyone posing that they are professionals in that field. Also, do not hesitate to do research online and compare notes. From there, you will be able to come back with something that works for you.

Surround yourself with a support system

The support system may include your family, colleagues, friends, or social net- works. These groups of amazing people may encourage and support you to meet your long-term goal. After you include them in your plan, they will feel accepted, offer opinions, and check on your progress. Analyze how things are going and en- courage you to continue taking a little break when necessary.

Your support system should include professionals in the field who will give sound advice and offer needed support and care.

CHAPTER 4

GASTRIC BAND HYPNOSIS: BENEFITS FOR WEIGHT LOSS AND HELP HEALING

Define and stamp permanently at the forefront of your thoughts, a mental image of yourself as succeeding. Hold this image tenaciously. Never grant it to blur. Your mind will try to build up the picture. Try not to develop deterrents in your creative mind. - Dr. Norman Vincent Peale

What can you practically expect in terms of improving your health and well- being? The facts demonstrate that some band patients experience reduced or total disappearance of high blood pressure, sleep apnea, and other incapacitating ailments. They can conceivably encounter the changeless reduction of different sicknesses, for example, diabetes. However, exactly how could that be? Also, how do well-being enhancements with the hypnotic gastric band contrast those of other weight loss programs? Let's find out.

Elements That Influence the Improvement of Your Health

Patients search out various weight loss procedures for several reasons. However, I would say it is health concerns that fat people might be insightful in considering weight reduction medical procedures. The goal ought to be improved well-being, not weight reduction only for weight reduction. Simultaneously, most patients are reasonably worried about their well-being, dangers that generally go with strategies, such as gastric detour. It is the reason many pick the hypnotic gastric band as a lower-chance than other options. In any case, the question that must ask. What about the outcomes? Improved well-being following any bariatric activity relies upon various components. One of the most evident is the measure of weight loss. The rate of the weight reduction likewise can assume a job, and quicker isn't nearly better. There is no doubt that weight reduction following gastric detour is usually faster and more emotional than after the hypnotic gastric band. Those patients who experience gastric detour may have a snappier improvement in a portion of their medical issues than patients undergoing hypnotic gastric band and but they are, to some degree, bound to have the different problems identified with hunger. Following a gastric detour, patients may lose as much as 5 pounds every week or more. In general, they will lose most of their weight during the first half-year and afterward start to decrease. Likewise, they should take nutrient B12 consistently to avoid paleness since iron can't be used by the body to make red platelets without vitamin B12.

Hypnotic gastric band patients will, in general, lose most of their weight over a year or two at an increasingly slow rate, generally about a pound to a pound and a half for each week. They also should be on a high-protein diet; however, they usually experience less difficulty keeping up good food or appetite. Since the stomach does not avoid, they don't require vitamin B12 supplements. The two techniques offer very comparative weight reduction results when we look at the outcomes for more than three to five years. With weight reduction, both gastric detour and hypnotic gastric band patients can encounter noteworthy improvement in various medical conditions, including diabetes, hypertension, rest apnea, reflux, and different back and joint pains. A few patients keep on experiencing at least one of these conditions despite losing a significant amount of weight.

Improvement in Diabetes

Diabetes is a complicated metabolic sickness, described by issues with producing the typical sugar glucose. Numerous individuals, despite everything, allude to it as "sugar diabetes." The real medical term is diabetes mellitus, which separates this disease from another ailment, diabetes insipidus, a turmoil including abundance water loss through the kidneys. All in all, when individuals, including doctors, use the expression "diabetes," they are alluding to diabetes mellitus. Additionally, there are two types of diabetes mellitus, Type I and Type II. In both types, the essential issue includes glucose levels in the circulatory system that are altogether higher than they ought to be. Type I diabetes has generally call adolescents beginning diabetes or inherited diabetes since it regularly happens in more youthful patients and will, in general, run in families. As of late, the name has been changed to Type I diabetes, because not all patients are youthful, nor do they have a family ancestry of the disease. This type of diabetes is affected somewhat by obesity, and large patients with type I disease can get slimmer. Type I patients all require insulin, either by infusion or by being naturally hungry. Type II diabetes is the more typical variety (90-95 percent) and is most closely related to obesity. This type of diabetes, Type II, will be the subject of the rest of this dialog. Insulin, a substance created by specific cells in the pancreas, encourages that procedure. Patients who have diabetes cannot produce glucose quickly. A straightforward method to comprehend diabetes is to consider insufficient insulin or feel that the insulin present is not viable because the cells have gotten impervious. In either case, more glucose stays in the circulatory system since less take-up by the cells. This procedure is significantly more confusing, but for purposes of our discussion, it will do. The relationship between obesity and diabetes is interesting, but the exact instrument by which obesity appears to "cause" diabetes isn't comprehended. If you are diagnosed with diabetes or even pre-diabetes, one of the main things your doc- tor will let you know is that you have to get in shape. So, by and by, we return to the issue of willful weight reduction. Pre-diabetes is essentially characterized as having higher-than-normal blood glucose levels, but not sufficiently high to meet the condition's criteria to be called diabetes.

The determination of Type II diabetes flags the beginning of a race to control this severe disease before it has time to cause any of the well-perceived pathologic effects. Likewise, high on the list of diabetes issues are coronary corridor disease and cerebral vascular disease, respiratory failure, and stroke being the primary sources of death among diabetes patients. The effects of fringe vascular disease, including potential appendage loss, are known to be significantly quickened by diabetes. Diabetes likewise meddles with nerve work, causing what is called diabetic neuropathy. It is the fundamental reason for impairing diabetic foot ulcers. Also, it perceives that individuals with diabetes don't have good white blood cell production to combat simple illnesses.

They commonly don't recuperate wounds or minor injuries just as those without diabetes. The primary concern is this: you have to get your diabetes leveled out because some terrible things will probably occur If you don't. Diabetes is a big issue and has been on the ascent in the United States for a few decades. Of course, this expansion matches the rise of obesity in our general public.

They won't have to take a prescription except if or until their glucose begins to return up. I have the screen the sugars intently once they return home, and most are shocked at how very much controlled they get better on the postoperative eating routine. That isn't the case with each patient, particularly the individuals who are on insulin, be that as it may, even patients on insulin will quite often need to re- duce their weight measurements. Longer-term, the outcomes following the hypnotic gastric band in patients with diabetes are amazingly encouraging. However, they rely upon a method aimed at the responsibility of an adjustment in the way of life. Notwithstanding weight reduction, getting exercise, and following a sound eating routine are fundamental parts of diabetes treatment.

CHAPTER 5

USEFUL TECHNIQUES FOR WEIGHT LOSS HYPNOSIS COULD INCLUDE:

It is enhancing confidence. Good suggestions can enable your feelings of confi- dence via speech that is inviting. Allergic Success. You might ask to envision fulfilling your weight reduction objectives and picture how it makes you feel through exercise. We are tapping the unconscious. From the hypnotic state, you might start to encounter the subconscious patterns that lead to lousy eating. On the flip side, you're inclined to be conscious of why we're making unhealthy food choices and portion control and set more careful approaches for making dishes decisions. They are fending off stress. Hypnotic tips can make it possible for you to tame your fear of not attaining weight loss success. Anxiety isn't any. One reason people may never begin in the very first available website. You are assessing and Reframing Habit Patterns. Once in mediation, you can analyze and study approaches you use intake and "turn off" those automated answers. We can start to slow down through repeated optimistic projections and thoroughly eliminate the automatic, subconscious thought. I am growing New Coping Mechanisms. Throughout hypnosis, it is possible to place much healthier ways to care for stress, relationships, and feelings. You may ask to imagine a stressful place and envision yourself reacting with a wholesome snack. You are rehearsing Healthy Eating. During exercise, you might ask to rehearse making healthy eating decisions, i.e., becoming ok with carrying food at a grocery store. It helps these healthy options to be automatic. Rehearsal might also be valuable for controlling cravings. You are making Better Food Choices. You may want and enjoy foods that are unhealthy. Hypnosis can help you begin to think about preference or taste for good chances, in addition to altering the portion sizes that you select. You are growing Unconscious Indicators. You might have discovered to detect the signals your body sends after you are feeling full during reproduction. Hypnotherapy can allow you to know about these indicators. Maybe not every proposal will apply to you. Suppose you are dealing with a hypnotherapist or self-hypnosis. In that case, your hypnotherapy strategy may include food recommendations; for example, Anne could function as instructing the subconscious to impede its automatic answers and provide the subconscious using new, more practical procedures to control anxiety. Addressing a certified hypnotherapist can help you improve your strategy to be specific to your requirements.

How Hypnotherapy Can Help You Attain Weight Loss

From the hypnotic state, your brain is much more responsive to trick. Many different studies have shown some exciting changes in your head through child- birth, which allows one to comprehend without thinking seriously about the info you are becoming. On the other side, you detach from a stunning mind. Thus, when you get pre- conceived thoughts, the clear conscious mind does not question what you hear. And in short, is how hypnosis can help you break down the barriers that keep you from losing weight. But repetition is very critical for success. That's the main reason a fantastic deal of hypnotherapists provides you home utilizing self-hypnosis records after a first trip. The barriers to your head are substantial. Only through repeated purpose will you powerful untangle and reframe those convictions. But hearing recurrent approaches and positive ideas about healthy eating is step one to the weight loss journey. You are teaching your brain to feel different. But these affirmations can help you to: Control Cravings Some weight loss hypnosis approaches let you get to that. For example, you may ask to picture sending off your cravings—say on a boat out to sea. Tips can also let you loosen your passions and discover how to handle them efficiently.

Anticipate Success Expectation requests details. The moment we anticipate success, we're more vulnerable to take into account the actions required to achieve that success. Weight loss hypnosis may plant the seed of success on your mind, and it's a clear subconscious incentive to keep you. Exercise Positivity Slimming down is often despised by negativity. You will observe that the foods that you "cannot" eat. Spicy foods are "murdering" you. Hypnotherapy enables people to plagiarize these ideas using a more favorable gentle—you are not depriving yourself; you are shedding what you do not need. Prepare Relapse we educate to believe that relapses are black—motives to supply up. However, hypnosis asks us to consider degeneration differently. A deterioration becomes a chance to examine what went wrong, learn from it, and be all set for temptation. Alter Your Behavior Enormous goals are attained one little step at the same moment. Hypnotherapy enables us to make minor alterations that nourish more prominent targets. Say you wind up with salty, salty foods through hypnosis; you can focus on picking a much healthier reward. Picture Success Ultimately, hypnotic visualization is a powerful incentive. Visualization allows you to "see" results and discover more about how that makes you feel. You may also envision your future-self telling you that you have what it takes to be successful.

CHAPTER 6

SWIMMING AND ITS CONTRIBUTIONS TO WEIGHT LOSS

World Health Organization (WHO) experts recommend routine physical activity to improve safety and well-being. Doctors also say regular exercise or playing sports is highly beneficial. While moving the body to improve health, lose weight, and feel better, it's essential to choose a fun activity to get the most out of it. Dancing, dancing, jogging, and swimming are the most popular choices.

Swimming promotes health and wellness

Swimming is a complete sport. It helps improve specific skills, lose weight, tone the body, and contribute to mental health. Therefore, many people are encouraged to practice it often, as part of their routine. It is considered an aerobic exercise since it requires large amounts of oxygen for the muscles' work, developing lung capacity. Among the best-known benefits of swimming are the release of emotional stress and tension, increased muscle tone, and the cardiovascular system's strengthening?

Know The Benefits Of Swimming To Jump Into The Water

1. Helps you lose weight while swimming, many of your muscles participate in the exercise, making it even more complete than walking. A comparative study concluded that swimming helped lose more weight than walking in sedentary older women. When measuring the reaction at the same intensity in each type of exercise per- formed three times a week, it found that the women who swam lost 1.1 kilograms and 2 centimeters more than those who limited themselves to walking. On the other hand, it observes that the risk of suffering knee and ankle injuries decreases with swimming.

2. It practice from an early age

Swimming is a sport that can be practiced from an early age, taking into ac- count some precautions, of course. Practicing it from 4-6 years of age can undoubtedly be very advantageous, but it is unnecessary to age the sport in any case.

3. Relax In this sense, swimming is no exception.

Take the test and see for yourself! Psychological experts indicate that swimming helps increase emotional intelligence, which contributes to mental health.

4. It is also useful in rehabilitation processes

The human body's density is similar to that of water, so the water supports the body, and the joints and the bones receive less impact. Swimming frequently uses in the rehabilitation process for specific injuries.

5. Improve the silhouette

By swimming, you can improve and correct your posture, in addition to developing good muscular resistance. It also helps to lose weight and keep it healthy, according to our body mass index.

6. Develops lung capacity

Swimming highly recommends in case of chronic respiratory diseases such as asthma. This exercise teaches us to keep pace with our breathing and improve oxy- gen uptake.

CHAPTER 7

SLEEPING BETTER: MAKING YOUR BODY LIGHT

In every one of the Hypno Slim sessions, I additionally utilize a ground-breaking sleep-inducing process that I have by and by created and called Creating Your Light Body. This procedure urges you to relinquish all your undesirable considerations, pictures, pictures, and profound cell recollections to identify with your weight and identify with nourishment. In mending these pictures, I utilize the representation of light to assist you with making another light body; a body that capacities in flawless agreement, so your digestion and each cell inside your bodywork immaculate well- being. The more significant part of your Hypno Slim sessions incorporates in any event called Creating Your Light Body. This procedure is also rehashed twice for the most extreme impact.

The Ultimate Hypno Slim Program incorporates eight Hypnosis chronicles, in addition to intuitive warm-up works out.

1. Intuitive Warm-up Exercises

These activities intend to heat your subliminal personality before you start tuning in to your Hypno Slim session. Your subconscious nature is the part of our thinking that will break through your review in your hypnotherapy session; this is the fantasy brain, enabling you to make a breakthrough, constructive and lasting changes to your feelings and behavior. Changes that will push you to all the more effectively, and that's only the tip of the iceberg, make your optimal immaculate body easy.

2. Unadulterated Motivation

The most significant piece of any effective, enduring change is an inspiration. At the point when we hear "change," our mind opposes typically – it's a piece of our body science and not something we can without much of a stretch warms up. That states, this hypnotherapy session will revamp your body's intuitive response to change. Lastly, bond all the fundamental strides to make you wake up and state, "this is the day I venture out arriving at my weight reduction objectives!"

3. Passionate Eating

For a considerable lot of us managing weight issues, bogus hunger is a huge issue. It's easy for a thin person to say, "Don't eat at all!" However, when your body has finished drinking a sugar-filled, bubbly drink or euphoric chocolate bar, you will feel how energetic and full of life you think – it's hard not to allow yourself to destroy everything! This session will focus on wiping out those bogus food cravings and educating your body on the best way to eat how you were destined to – eating when you're eager and eating for sustenance. How much better do you feel when you've completed that chocolate bar or a pack of chips? It is the ideal opportunity to discharge all the old psychological weight that has made you clutch your abundance weight. Over and over, I have seen tremendous and positive changes happen due to this session. I would need to state this is one of the most dominant sessions of the whole program.

4. Gastric Band

This session offers a progressive new thought in the fascinating clinical field. Similarly, like a gastric band, the medical procedure takes out an abundance of weight through substantial alteration – gastric band hypnotherapy works at the intuitive level to assist you with thinning down step by step, aside from the cost, healing, and symptoms.

Gastric band trance demonstrates to create the equivalent and once in a while preferred results over gastric band medical procedure – without the medical process. It may appear to be trying to accept, yet this shows precisely how great trance can be with changing conduct and shedding pounds. In this mesmerizing, I utilize explicit systems to retrain your cerebrum in ways that leave it persuaded you have experienced specific medical procedures and that you have a real gastric band setup. The consequence of this hypnotherapy approach mirrors the aftereffect of the medical system. You feel full more rapidly, which encourages you to abstain from indulging.

5. Altering the Band

Likewise, with its carefully embedded partner, a hypnotherapy-based gastric band additionally should be balanced. Fortunately, it won't require a touch of cut- ting, testing, or join and, once more, is altogether done in the brain. I'll tell your psyche precisely the best way to imagine the band altering. Your weight keeps changing, and your frame of mind toward nourishment movements to a reliable equalization of control and sustenance. Let my words manage your psyche into a profound, loosened state, so all recommendations are met with zero opposition, and the gastric band can work freely to assist you with getting more fit quickly.

6. Good dieting

Longings are your body's method for attempting to get something it most likely shouldn't have (like refined carbs, salt, synthetic substances, handled nourishment, etc.). It's so used to getting what it needs, at whatever point it needs that, similar to a grumpy baby, it will attempt to pitch a fit. It does this not by shouting and beating on the floor but by flooding your brain with pictures, scents, tastes, and a persistent want to make you yield. Be that as it may, with this hypnotherapy session, you'll not exclusively have the option to step your longings into the ground, yet besides supplant those yearnings with reliable other options. You may not feel that grapes could fill in for chips – however, with the privilege of guided words and feelings saturating your psyche, they will.

7. Exercise Motivator

Indeed, I'm going to state it; the feared 'E' word. A significant piece of any effective get-healthy plan includes venturing up your degree of physical movement.   Let's be honest. When you return home after a monotonous work, cook, en- courage your family, pack things, and prepare– the exact opposite is to exercise. With the intensity of hypnotherapy, you can build your craving and assurance to practice every day. Envision how refreshing you will feel when you step up every morning with the longing to move your body in some reliable manner. When in any event, hearing, thinking, or seeing the word practice propels you to your very center.

8. Reward SESSION Think Yourself Thin

The more you envision yourself as the slim individual you want to be, the more rapidly this will end up being your world. In this free mesmerizing chronicle, you will utilize the intensity of your intuitive personality to wash away indeed your abundance fat and make your optimal flawless body.

9. Reward SESSION Boost Your Metabolism

Your ground-breaking intuitive personality controls your body's oblivious procedures, such as managing your pulse and breathing rate. In this free trance recording, you will go into your brain's control room to enhance your digestion and assume back responsibility for your body. Here are some great/life viable instances of Hypnotherapy related by some trance inducer for weight control: Mary came to me since she needed to get more fit, besides, since she was feeling so wild that she wasn't getting a charge out of any piece of her life any longer. She is examining the legitimacy of her reality-monotonous routine, that is, working hard to do business in a job she is not valued. She strives to make money and gets along well with her essential people. Despite this, the relationship is excellent but not unique and has been trying. Anyway, she lost more than 100 pounds during most of her 30s. Mary was an ordinary customer in that she had a go at everything alone to shed pounds that she could think about that appeared to be sensitive to her. There is unquestionably no deficiency of weight reduction plans and projects to be on, and she had attempted every one of them. She realized how to shed pounds. Be that as it may, she generally recovered it. What's more, she was burnt out on intuition about it to such an extent. She was baffled about attempting to "fathom" this issue and investing such a large amount of her energy committed to this one part of her life that appeared to have been as long as she can remember center. Mary is excellent at her particular employment and knows how to issue settle. She's fruitful in basically every other part of her life, yet this a specific something, losing the weight, just evaded her. It generally had. Furthermore, she was so baffled and tired that she didn't have the foggiest idea, whether it was worth any event or attempting any longer.

CHAPTER 8

HOW TO LOSE WEIGHT FAST WITHOUT WORKING OUT?

There are so many different options; it is natural to doubt this, but what if I can show you an effective method? Are you interleaved in discovering the secret to losing weight quickly that the Hollywood elites have been hiding for years? Regardless of the plan, is one of the millions of people tired of not being able to lose weight? I will share with you a secret that is not common knowledge, and few people know. Here are ways to lose weight without workout:

Modifying Your Diet for Weight Loss

If you are a person who consumes food because of emotional or spiritual problems, then you need to have these issues addressed. You will be able to make very little progress with your weight loss if there is an underlying issue. Many people also eat when they are experiencing times of stress. You must learn to modify these habits also. Various diets and weight loss programs promise delivery of quick weight loss. However, most crash diets are unhealthy. They strip the body of water weight and muscle tissue. These are two key ingredients that the body needs when it comes to burning body fat. With a crash diet, you may see an initially massive loss of weight on the outset. Your body will eventually send itself into starvation mode when it realizes it is not getting the appropriate amount of nutrients and food. With your metabolism in starvation mode, it becomes increasingly difficult to lose weight. It is the point where most people abandon their diets altogether. To lose weight permanently, you prepare to modify your food intake. Do you know why most dieting methods are ineffective? Unfortunately, these programs attempt to do too much, nearly pulling and pushing your body, eradicating any chance of success; what happens when you try to push and pull something simultaneously? Simply, nothing at all, opposing forces in different directions cancel out their energies. While this example may seem silly, this illustrates what effect most dieting programs have on your body and why they always fail.

There are two fundamental maxims you will need to do:

- Reduce your daily calorie intake.

- Burn off your body's fat reserves.

However, these two concepts are actually at odds with one another. If you choose to reduce your daily caloric intake, your body begins to burn less fat. Un- fortunately, this is how our body copes. It is a survival mechanism that kicks on to help guard against dangerous circumstances, such as famine.

Maintaining Your Weight Loss

A few months after becoming a member of the weight-loss club, you have experienced the so-called weight loss success, and when you stopped taking regular exercise, she regained the weight loss effect. It seems as if it is almost like a plot to keep you paying to keep on going to the slimming club; otherwise, you find that you can't maintain your weight loss. So, to maintain the success you feel you've added, you need to do more than just regularly go to a slimming club or follow a diet in a newspaper. It's about changing your mindset about your weight and realizing that diets on their work. Yes, if you follow what writes, or what you tell and lose some weight. However, the value is in many, and most cases regained very quickly once you decide you're going back to a "normal" diet. If diets don't work, then what can you do to be the way that you would like to be, and be healthy too eat regularly: You may have tried to lose weight by skipping meals entirely. It doesn't work because your blood sugar level drops, and you begin to crave lots of sugar and other simple carbohydrates. As a result, he will probably find yourself overeating high calorie, high fat, unhealthy food, and, see it anyway, kudos goes back on very quickly. Healthy diet: If you consider what you eat and try to make your diet as healthy as possible without being fanatical, you will have a greater chance of controlling your weight by controlling your mindset. A healthy diet means a balanced diet, eating more fresh fruits and vegetables, low-fat protein, healthy fats (such as olive oil and avocado), and lots of complex carbohydrates. It also means cutting right down on food containing sugar and white foods such as white flour, white rice, and white pasta and eating instead more whole-meal foods Relax frequently: If you tend to eat more when you feel stressed, wait for a while and think that the pressure is gradually increasing to close your eyes and relax your breath while breathing and relieve stress. Listen to your body: Learn to listen to what your body tells you about your needs at any time of the day, and let yourself have whatever you seem to need, even if you understand the health guidelines above.

Get enough sleep for weight loss

When we think of the most important things that our bodies need, sleep is right up there with food, water, and oxygen; the amount of sleep you get daily can dramatically affect your health and weight. But do we know how must sleep we need? As a general guide, most adults should be aiming to get around 7 - 8 hours a day. Our bodies are different. Some people may find that their sleep time peaks at 6 hours a day, while others may need about 9 hours. Sleep deprivation, however, is a big problem, and if you are only managing around 4-5 hours a night, then your body is being deprived of sleep.

Let's firstly look at the benefits of getting a good night sleep: Sleep Naturally Repairs Your Body: Extra protein molecules produce while sleeping, which helps fight infection, and your immune system repairs cells. Sleep Reduces Stress Levels: A good quality sleep can help lower blood pressure and levels of stress hormones in your body. Greater Concentration: A good night's sleep will allow you to concentrate better the following day and aid memory function. More Relaxed: A good sleep will mean you wake up more refreshed and relaxed. If you don't get enough sleep regularly, all of the above benefits offsets. So, this may mean waking up emotion groggy, emotion more stressed, and unable to concentrate. You will also be more prone to illness and higher blood pressure. You may think that being deprived of sleep and emotion tired may result in a loss of appetite and weight loss, but the truth is that a lack of sleep may lead to weight gain. Sleep helps keep in check the hormones in your body that control your appetite, so if you are not getting enough sleep, your need will increase, and you will feel even hungrier. Sleep deprivation will cause your body to have reduced energy levels, and your body will crave high-fat content foods that may give you a temporary boost. These foods tend to be high in calories and salt or sugar; they will not fill you up because they lack nutrition and will leave you sluggish and hungry again very soon. Nothing will set you better for the day than a sound refreshing sleep followed by a well-balanced breakfast. To aid your sleep, try to limit your consumption of alcohol and spicy foods. Try and unwind naturally before bed with a nice long soak or some relaxation exercises. Try to avoid using alcohol as your primary way of relaxing and relieving stress. If you are looking to lose weight, as well as eating a sensible and balanced diet and taking regular exercise, you need to be getting a good night's sleep every night.

CHAPTER 9

WHAT FOODS SHOULD I AVOID?

When you are going on any kind of diet, it is essential to make sure that you are avoiding the right foods. That is why we will spend some time looking at the foods that we should avoid when it comes to the fat-burning diet and the foods we should avoid when it comes to the low carb diet. Putting these two together and learning what foods are good for us and which ones we need to avoid can make all of the difference in the health benefits that we can get.

Foods to Avoid on the Fat Burning Diet

The first part that we will take a look at here is some of the foods you can work with when it comes to the fat-burning diet. To start, even though carbs are allowed on this diet plan, you do need to be careful about the kinds of carbs that you are eating. You want to focus on this diet with lots of whole grains, whether that is bread or pasta, and you get lots of healthy fruits and vegetables. However, you need to avoid a few types of foods during this time, especially if you are on one of the lower-carb diets. In some of these, you need to avoid things like white and processed carbs. That means the white pieces of bread and kinds of pasta, and the baked goods and sweets are all things that we need to avoid when we go through this kind of diet plan. Stick with the healthier options, and you will do a lot better when you are on this diet plan. Another thing to cut out is processed and fast foods. Sure, this taste amazing and can make life a little bit easier when it comes down to the busy nights with your family. But when you are working on losing weight and improving your health, and when you are on the fat burning diet, these are things that you need to avoid. Make sure that you are cutting these out as much as possible, and if you can, con- sider just not having them at all. The beverages that you are allowed to have on this kind of diet plan will vary as well. Things like water, tea, and milk are the best choices for you to have. You can have a few fruit juices on occasion, but make sure that they don't come with a bunch of bad things or extra sugars in them and consider watering them down to make them a bit better as well. You want to make sure that you are as hydrated as possible, and avoid things like sodas and pops and all of the sports drinks and other things that will ruin your health. Remember, both the fat burning diet and the low carb diet are all about helping you eat healthier and wholesome foods for the whole body. Doing so will ensure that you are prepared for success and can lose the weight you want while also improving other health aspects. If you are not careful about some of the foods you are consuming and eat the bad ones for your body, you will not get the right health you need.

Low Carb Diet Foods to Avoid

You will find many similarities in foods that you should avoid between these two diets, making them even easier to follow when you go through and use them well. The low carb diet is often more restrictive than some other options, so we need to keep that in mind.   The first type of food that we need to avoid is the grains and the slices of bread. Throughout the world, a meal will be a typical food that many cultures like to eat. We can enjoy many types of bread, but the carbohydrate content will be high in many cases. Both the food that manufactures with refined sugars and the whole- grain bread will be more top in carbs, and when you are on this kind of diet, you will need to cut down on these because they are likely to hold onto way more carbs than you are supposed to eat during the day.   You also need to pay attention to the amount of fruit you eat. While this is not entirely off the table, you may find a few types of fruits that do not recommend because they will come with the higher carbs content. Sweet and dried fruits are going to be the biggest culprits here. For example, having about .25 cup of dates will be somewhere between 20 and 33 grams of carbs, but a small banana would have closer to 18 grams.   Most vegetables will be fine in moderation, but we need to worry about some of the starchy vegetables we are eating. The majority of the herbs that we will want to eat will come with higher fiber content, which helps us control some of our blood sugars and weight loss levels. But this will not extend to all the vegetables we are looking for. Some of the herbs considered starches will contain more carbs than fibers, so we need to limit them as much as possible on this kind of diet plan. There are many great vegetables that you can enjoy when it comes to being on a low carb diet, and you can enjoy them as long as you monitor your carb intake. Some of the vegetables you need to watch out for because of the carb content will include beets, yams, sweet potatoes, potatoes, and corn. Some of the better options you can work with and provide you with fewer carbs and more nutrients will include mushrooms, lettuce, cauliflower, avocados, spinach, and green beans. There are also a few other grains that we need to watch out for when we are working with the low carb diet. Even though there are many pasta types, we have to be careful, and using pasta is not expensive. It will go with many carbs in it, though, which is not suitable for this kind of diet plan. You will find that a cup of pasta cooked will be nearly 40 grams of carbs, and whole wheat is only slightly better with 31 grams of carbs. The best alternative you can use in your meals for this one is spiralized vegetables or shirataki noodles. Cereal should avoid, as well. Most of these will be full of sugar, and that will not do you any favors when working with the low carb diet. You will also find that oatmeal generally considers better and healthier than other oatmeal, but it still brings 28 grams of carbohydrates, which we need to worry about. It is one of the biggest mistakes that you can make on this kind of diet plan. Yes, the liquid will come in with a few nutrients that we can work with, but there are a ton of carbs and sugars that we need to deal with, which will cause a massive in- crease in our levels of blood sugars along the way. For example, there are upwards of 48 grams of carbs found in every 12 ounces of unsweetened apple juice. A bottle of regular soda is only going to come in with 39 grams in comparison. And it gets worse. If you are working with that same size but in grape juice, there could be up to 60 grams of carbs, which is already above what most low carb diets will allow you for the whole day. These are going to provide us with a ton of nutritional benefits that are so good for us. These legumes and beans are going to come with high fiber content, and they are great at helping with heart complications and inflammation. However, we have to remember that they are going to have a higher amount of carbs. It doesn't mean that we need to get rid of the legumes and the beans thoroughly. It is often going to depend on what we are doing for the rest of the day. De- pending on how many carbs you have in a day, or plan to have, you may eat a small amount of these legumes and beans. But you need to plan it all out and be careful in the process. And finally, we are going to need to be careful about the milk that we consume. If you would like to get some of the right nutrients that your body needs, like the B vitamins, calcium, and potassium, we need to make sure that we drink milk. But when we are on a low carb diet, it is often best to go with a plant-based option or something else. It is because an eight-ounce serving of milk will come in with 12 to 13 grams of carbs that we need to worry about, and that is never a good thing. As we can see with both of these diet plans, there are many things that we will need to limit ourselves on and that we are not allowed to have in the first place any longer. It can make it hard to follow this kind of diet plan and cut down on what we can consume. But the good news is that it does provide us with delicious and nutritious food that we can enjoy, which is always a good thing. Ensure that before you get started on this kind of eating plan for some of your own needs.

CHAPTER 10

10 WEIGHT LOSS MYTHS

The myths are the highest misconceptions I have found in my 15 years as a professional trainer. Use them immediately in your daily routine. To have success, you have to have the right information, but you will also need the determination and motivation. You hold power in you to get started now.

Myth 1- If I work out with weights, I will get big and bulky

The only way to get big and fat is to continue to have bad eating habits. You need to find your resting metabolism. How much food do you need to consume to be healthy, lose weight, and feel great? You have to try hard on any person to get your muscles to grow. It is the last thing to worry about. Focus on using a set of muscles a day to work out to burn the maximum number of calories. A recovered power will always outperform a tired muscle. That means fewer calories burned for you if your passion is exhausted.

Myth 2- Just doing cardio will give me the best fat burning result.

Although cardio stands for heart lungs, it does not mean the most potent fat burner. The harder you push your body in one sitting or workout with the same exercise, the more likely you are to use your muscle tissue for energy versus fat stores. Look at fat burning in the 3-day window. Not today, even if that program worked, the biggest downside would be that your lungs expand to a new level EVERY 10 minutes. That means from the very first day, you start losing your ability to burn as much fat. Suppose you can't figure out why you have skinny legs. It could be from too much running. That may crash your metabolism. How long can you be a marathon runner? Some may try, but at the same time, it is not very likely you. We talk 50 miles a week! I am not against the long-term. It is not my entire game plan; it feels good.

Myth 3- You need to work your whole body every day

Your body needs time to adjust. Your body does all of its replacing and drop- ping while you are asleep. Around 90% of any result happens when you are sleeping. Not when you are awake. Your body will adapt to any exercise you do every day. Fast adaptation will warrantless results. You want to pick a large and small muscle group per day. Attack it with a lot of energy. Wash and repeat that process weekly. When you come back weekly, you will be more robust—giving you a better fat burning workout each time. Too much overtraining happens when you do the same muscles or exercises every day.

Myth 4- Liposuction will give me the answer I need

The fact is, you will most likely be back to the beginning. What? How is that? Well, your plastic surgeon can only take off so much at one time. Most of the time, that magic number is a WHOPPING ten pounds. After your surgery, you can't move for three weeks. I do not care what they tell you. I have seen it over and over. Since you can't do anything, your body slows down. So, anything you eat stays with you. I have seen people gain weight. Not to mention that you have rub or massage your bruises, so water does not get trapped between your skin.

Myth 5- Fat is bad for me

The fact is fat has two meanings. One is the kind you eat. That has a few dif- ferent names within that. Then their body fat. Cells or adipose tissue. They are not the same. Your body fat stores in food. With maybe some water. End of question. Dietary fat has taken a bad rap. In my eyes and 15 years of experience-fat is not even our problem with our foods. You will need fat in your body if you do not want to age quickly, or you want to drop body fat, keep hormone levels balanced out, re- pair muscles. Otherwise, your body is missing some pieces of the puzzle. It is not balanced. It does, without any doubt, carry more calories per gram than the other significant macronutrients. They are the carbs and proteins.

Myth 6- All carbohydrates are bad for me

You will need them to balance your blood sugars. Which is the key to dropping body fat and energy? Not mention not feeling depressed. If you do a no-carb or ketogenic diet, you will quickly find out what it's like to feel like dirt without carbs. You don't have to do this! Always know how your food harvests. Then what happens on each stop of its way to your table. If it was originally brown and now it is white, something is missing. To the body, it is not the same food anymore. The name of the food does not matter. Your body breaks food down. It can be called wheat bread, even have colored added to the bread, and processed and bleached. It is not the same; real wheat will not cause weight gain. It will not cause weight gain. Processed weight will almost always cause weight gain. Are you starting to see the picture?

Myth 7- Rice, wheat, and grains are bad

It does not matter the kind of food it is. It matters what happens to the blood sugar once you eat the food. The average consumer buys food that is broken down already or is using sugar for a preservative. The two hot diets out Paleo and raw vegan neither eat any kind of processed food. Let the light flash for a minute. Ok. Brown rice is your friend as long as it is not instant.

Myth 8- Red meat is terrible for me

It is what the meat process in is what is bad for you. Maybe it has been pumped full of hormones. When you add white processed bread to a heavily processed fat, that's your combination for a heart attack. The absolute highest food in vitamin A is red meat liver. A burger from the fast-food place can get you in trouble—it processes in all ways and preserves and over-processed.

Myth 9- Your metabolism is slow

That is another word that has multiple meanings. Your metabolism is your ability to break your food down. Storing your food is another process. The slower the food breaks down, the less chance to keep that food or call it energy. Most likely, your body breaks down food, OK. Honestly, I have never seen a real case where your body does not break the food down correctly. Other situations may cause issues. When someone messes with your hormones that can have a dramatic effect on weight. Just at all costs, stay away from messing around with hormones. Your body will become different at that point. More importantly, you may always be stuck taking that hormone or thyroid medication.

Myth 10- I only need to focus on my calorie intake.

Yes, the amount of food you consume does affect your ability to lose fat. The kinds of food are just as important, if not more important. What your body does with the food once it is inside you is the real question. Can your body burn this food up, or does your body need to repair it? If, not it will store. I have seen first- hand when a person gets a lap band and get great results—eating less than 1000 calories a day. Then after a couple of months, the body adapts to that 1000 calories. Now, what are you going to do? A lap band is a band around your stomach that is surgically put there. It shuts off your signals to want to eat. It makes your stomach smaller. Make sure you put the kind of foods before how much of food. Surround yourself with the proper types of food.

CHAPTER 11
WORKOUT

How To Boost Your Motivation To Work Out?

There are two significant components of weight loss; your diet and your daily activities. Keeping an active lifestyle will increase your metabolic rate. It will make your body burn more energy even when you are resting.   To integrate workouts into your lifestyle, you should make sure that you enjoy them. If it feels too much like work, it will be too difficult to maintain. There will come a time that the distractions and temptations around you will defeat your mind.

How To Build Motivation For Working Out?

Before you can start lifting weights, jogging, or doing other activities, you should put in writing what you want to achieve. If you're going to lose weight, you should set the exact number of pounds you want to lose and the amount of time you have to achieve your goal. You could also put your dreams on specific body parts like your waistline or your arms. Following the S.M.A.R.T. philosophy to set goals is an ideal tool to use. It ensures goals are Specific, Measurable, Attainable, Realistic, and have a Timeline. You should then find a workout plan that fits your schedule and your personality. You should consider the time you have for your workouts and the effort you can devote to it.

Remind Yourself Of The Benefits Of Working Out

Being aware of the benefits of working out will help you continue to do it. You can also build your willpower and avoid laziness. It will remind you that you are not doing this just to look great and become healthier.

List Your Favorite Activities

If you love dancing, you should include that in your workout plan. If you prefer sports, you should train for the sport you want to participate in. By doing things that you like, you will transition to an active lifestyle with much more ease. Include various activities in your exercise plan besides doing what you love, you should also make it a habit to try new things and vary your workout plan activities. Lifting weights or running all the time will be- come boring after some time. If your body does not present with a challenge every time, it will no longer improve.

Prepare The Necessary Equipment And Outfits

Spending for your workout plan is like investing in your body; you will be expecting a return on your investment. Not only will you feel like an athlete, but this will make you work harder and become more disciplined in following your strategies.

Make Your Workouts A Social Activity

You should avoid doing everything by yourself. Just like in your diet plan, you should also include the people around you. Join people who also like to work out. Motivation, enthusiasm, and positive thinking are contagious. You will have a better chance of continuing your weight loss program if you have these people around.

Analyze The Factors That Motivate You

You should also use your metacognitive abilities to improve your performance. Every time you feel extra motivated, you should analyze the internal and external sources of your motivation. Understanding these factors will give you a deeper understanding of your way of thinking. You can use some of these factors to stimulate your inspiration when you are feeling down.

Reward Yourself For Reaching Your Goals

Rewards are things that you allow yourself to have when you reach a specific goal. They expect to increase the likelihood that you will repeat you're positive behaviors. You should decide on the rewards that you will give yourself when making your goals. The thought of the prize will help motivate you. When the workout routine becomes hard, you should remind yourself of the reward, you will get if you push through. You should make sure. However, you will be able to follow through with your promise. The most important deposits are the ones that you give to yourself.

Recharge Your Motivation to Exercise

The only thing standing between you and your desired body is mental disorders, so to overcome those speed bumps and avoid the inevitable excuses, follow the top methods below to restart exercise and mental and emotional state. You Think – my scales are stuck, why am I bothering?

Rethink - This podge will go Stick with it. Weight loss is never consistent, and the scales, unless they are cheap or faulty, will never lie. First off, the more weight you have to lose, the quicker it will come out – IN THE BEGINNING. After that, it will all start to slow down. Most people reach a weight loss plateau, where they don't lose any weight for several weeks. One more important point – do not weigh yourself every day; it's a nasty habit. Your weight will rise and fall every day, but overall, it will drop. Weigh every week or every two weeks. That way, any loss in value is a much bigger motivator. Weighing yourself is the best way to demotivate yourself, so don't do it. Just because you aren't losing any pounds doesn't mean that your body isn't losing inches, and the only way to tell that is how your clothes fit. Give yourself plenty of credit for how much better you look and use that as your motivation to continue. Redo - Move your routine up a gear As you lose weight, your metabolism will alter to accommodate the lighter, smaller you. That means you will have to change how you encourage your body to burn fat and shed pounds. If you are already on a light diet of around 1500 calories a day, don't cut any more off. Instead, make your workouts more intense and work out for a bit longer each time. Not only will this result in more calories burn off, but it will also make your cardio capacity much larger. It means that you will find it easier to exercise and be motivated to work out for just that little longer. Increase the stationary bike's resistance, incline the treadmill more, walk longer than now, and walk faster or run once every minute. Between toning exercises, fit in a set of jumping jacks, running on the spot, or step-ups. You Think - I really can't manage another rep Rethink - Don't my biceps look fantastic! Suppose you need a motivational boost, a bit of a lift, psych yourself up men- tally and emotionally while you are training. It can increase your muscle power by up to 8% s well as the size, and bigger muscles result in an increase in metabolism, which burns off fat faster. So, if you needed just one bit of motivation, there it is. Mental imagery is a beautiful boost – when your arms or legs feel tired, imagine bigger and stronger muscles, tell yourself how great you look, and you will get another rep or two out. Redo – Take it down a notch If you really can manage another rep at the same rate, lighten things off a bit. If you are lifting weights, knock the values down by 10% until you know you can do another rep in good form. If you are sprinting circuits, slow it down for the last one. The more effort you put in, the better the return you can get. If you can't do it, then never beat yourself, but keep this in mind-pushing the limit further will get the result you never dream of. You Think - I can't run a mile! Rethink – That jogger looks like Brad Pitt/Angelina Jolie – whoever takes your fancy at the time! When you are slogging your way through that mile, turn your thinking to what is going on around you. You may slow down a little, but you will keep on going, and you will finish that mile. Repeat a mental mantra over and over again – something like "I am a running machine," and you will find that you can go for longer and further. Redo – Divide and Conquer If you are running a mile, split it up into some bits of running and some walk- ing. Jog for about a quarter of a mile, then jog for half a mile, and then do the final stretch. As you get better and fitter and leaner, you can fly for additional and gradually cut down the walking time. If you can do it three times a week, you can spend a whole week. Your motivation? Your fitness and how you look.

Think about how much better you feel, and you will keep on going. Do set up a routine for running, though. If you only go as and when it will not work. You Think - I've damaged my knee/leg/arm, etc., I won't be able to do any exercise for a month Rethink – Where did I put that Pilates DVD? If you injure yourself and stop working out, it takes a maximum of three days for your body to start losing its conditioning. If this is not enough to get you up and walk around, please tell yourself that there is more than one way to achieve your goals. List all negative thoughts first, then turn them into positive comments. For example, "I can't go to my exercise class tonight, everything I've done will all go to waste" turn into "oh well, now I can start using that Pilates DVD I bought." Redo – Switch things out .

CHAPTER 12

HEALTH AND FITNESS TIPS

1. To increase your muscle mass, raise weights twice a week. This muscle burns up more calories, even if you don't exercise. Go to the gym, buy a few values for home, go for a walk in your rucksack with a bottle of water, or go for a weighted workout.

2. Caring for your heart and lungs by remaining active for at least 30 minutes each day. It breaks down into more than one workout so that it might mean 2 x 15- minute walks.

3. Eat tiny quantities of healthy fats: avocado, fatty fish, olive/flax oil, nuts, and seeds; these will look after your back, lungs, and veins. Eat fewer BAD fats: fried food, beef, cookies, chocolate, chips, biscuits, butter, which will harm your cardio- vascular system and make you obese. Delete from your diet ALL hydrogenated fats; they are terrible for you and hidden in many ready-made cookies, pies, crisps, puddings, candy, chocolates ... These fats harm your health enormously. Avoiding them will help you avoid diets rich in calories, salt, sugar, and low nutrients. See labels.

4. Protein will make you feel full, and after exercise, it will help repair muscle. Seek to get protein from skinless chicken, tofu, pulses (beans and peas), and oily fish such as

salmon, fresh tuna, and mackerel; these also provide other beneficial ingredients and are low in weakly saturated fats.

5. Ensure your carbohydrate must eat; they enable you to work out and burn fat but eat SLOW BURN carbohydrates such as oats (porridge), brown bread rather than white, brown rice. If you want to reduce fat, then start replacing half of your carbohydrates with steamed vegetables at your evening meal.

6. Drink more water; the body often sends out the same thirst-signal as hunger. Drink water in the morning, and during the day, particularly during and after the exercise. Cut it on coffee and tea; avoid fizzy drinks.

7. Take a slice of fruit and drink water instead of drinking high-calorie, challenging to digest fruit juice.

8. Pay attention to sports drinks. A sports drink bottle may replace all the calories you have just burned in your activity unless you are training very hard. Put in a water bottle instead.

9. eep an eye on your beer! Alcohol is high in calories, and mixers are high.

10. Do not get hungry; that will lead you to eat the wrong things. Bring nutritious snacks everywhere you go; bananas, tomatoes, rice cakes, dried fruit, and nuts (though

they're easy to carry on). Boredom or a lack of stimulation can trigger hunger. Go around the garden for a walk or wander, or do the vacuuming. Eat five small meals a day instead of 3 big ones.

11. Look at the serving sizes; they're usually smaller than they ought to be. If a smaller portion leaves you hungry, add a giant spoon of steamed broccoli, cauliflower, or other vegetables.

12. Eat breakfast. Those who eat breakfasts lose more weight in experiments than people who don't. You can't work out effectively without feeding well to attain your capacity.

13. If you're hungry, don't go shopping. Write a list when you go, stick to it, and don't be tempted by exceptional food offers you know are bad for you.

14. Look at the contents in whatever you offer. Look at the total amount of fat and what kind of fat— avoid saturated fats and hydrogenated fats as they are associated with heart disease development. Look at the number of calories you will eat, and the amount of salt you will eat—the more additives on a label, in general, the less goodness in the food. If you have time to prepare some meals with fresh ingredients, you will improve your health and probably reduce fat, since most foods are high in fat and salt.

15. Do not fill the children's house with crisps, biscuits, and

sweets, it's not good for them, and it will encourage you to snack on them too. Try to move the whole family towards healthier eating; this will help prevent your children from obesity, heart disease, and diabetes when they are your age, giving them a long, quality life.

16. Stock up on good food. Write down a list of delicious healthy things you may have forgotten you love, and make sure your cupboards are full of them; cherry tomatoes, whole meal baked beans, kiwis, mangoes, and mar-mite.

17. Create the sandwich and get it to work. Buy whole-grain rolls and tins of salmon and tuna-make a sandwich and pick some fruit in just a few minutes. Even a sandwich shop will be full of fat and nutrient low. Hold on to the tuna mayo!

18. Watch less television: it will give you less incentive to nibble, more time to work out, or prepare yourself for the day after. The organization may be the key to healthier lifestyles.

19. Motivate yourself to alter your lifestyle and family. To the children, set an example that mum and dad are fit, active, and healthy. Take them on walks, ride a bike, walk to the shops, and swim. Take them to the local football, dance at the basketball fitness center. Our kids need our help to avoid the growing obesity epidemic, heart disease, diabetes, and other lifestyle-related diseases. Change their eating

GastricBand Hypnosis

habits; you are just going to do them good.

LEAD BY EXAMPLE.

20. Buy a video exercise to do at home, instead of watching television. Choose Yoga or Pilates, Aerobics or Roller for Relaxation. There is a vast range of offerings on offer; talk to me for help. Buy a balanced living journal for inspiration, tips, and learning workouts. There are four good ones: Zest, Men's Health, Super Fit, Health, and Fitness, buy yourself for ideas on a healthy meal or low-fat cookbook.

21. Remember to have some snacks and some enjoyment; life is for living, it should be nice to be safe, not work.

22. Slow down, stop rushing, get organized, and spend time cooking, exercising, and life in general.

23. Take some time to unwind and relax. To stay healthy, exercise, yoga, and Pilates can help you do this; you need to lower the stress levels, and so a warm can- dlelight bath can help.

24. Do exercise and eating healthy, a regular and pleasurable part of every day of your life. You will live longer, protect your children's health, and be a healthier, safer human.

CHAPTER 13

GASTRIC BAND HYPNOSIS FOR FOOD ADDICTION

Weight loss has turned into a noteworthy and over the top factor in today's society. With the numerous people following significant name trends to drop dress sites to fit into the attire scopes of such fashion icons like Kate Moss, losing weight should be done accurately else you could be taking a chance with your wellbeing and creating significant issues in the long-run and present

The step you have to take when losing weight is to examine what you need from it. Planning is a vital part of losing weight since this is the thing that develops your inspiration. So before beginning any eating regimen get pen and paper and record a few achievements that you can effectively accomplish. A decent start is gauging yourself, recording the weight down and afterward setting week by week target of 2.3lhs or monthly targets of 8-12lbs. Weight loss doesn't mean you will live the following 6-12 months torturing yourself with eating regimens and exercise. The hardest part of weight loss is adhering to it and taking care of business, 90% of people haul out before the end of their plan and end up putting the weight they lost hack on inside weeks. Keep in mind weight loss can be fun if you need it to he, meeting your monthly targets can give you a genuine feeling of achievement so treat yourself to something like another aroma to further add to yourself assurance, and if you are surpassing your targets, a rare sustenance treat won't hurt. This will provide all the assistance you need in keeping to your plan and helping you go the whole way to a superior life and an improved body

Overall, we get more fit to look great and feel good. The vast majority wet more fit in the springtime, and this is for a few reasons. Right off the hat, after the Christmas period, they may have gained a couple of pounds that they need to shed because they need to set themselves up for their mid year occasions where they will sunbathe on the shoreline in a piece of some swim shorts. The dread of several people seeing you in a semi stripped state will make you need to look as well as can be expected, so diet and exercise have a noteworthy influence on this

When all is said and done only the sheer vibe of having the option to fit inte garments that you never figured you could can truly transform you and your persona, and this is why we do it Why is it Hard to Control Your Diet?

It appears everybody nowadays is attempting to lose weight. We are modified by our condition to book, dress, and even act in a specific way.

Each time you get a magazine, turn on the TV or check out yourself, you are reminded of it. You start to hate your body losing control, disappointed, focused on, apprehensive, and now and again even discouraged.

If losing weight is tied in with eating fewer calories than your body needs and doing some activity to support your digestion, at that point why are such a significant number of individuals as yet attempting to lose weight?

Losing weight has to do with your considerations and convictions as much as it has to do with what you cat. Give me a chance to give you a model. You are staring at the TV, and an advertisement is shown demonstrating a chocolate cheddar cake that you can make utilizing just 3 fixings. You weren't hungry previously, however, since you have seen that cheddar cake you might feel denied and you need to cat. Your feelings are revealing to you that you have to eat, although your stomach isn't disclosing to you that you are hungry.

This is called passionate eating. It is our feelings that trigger our practices.

You may find that when you are feeling focused or depressed, you have this need to cat something since it solaces you somehow or another. The issue is that generally, it isn't healthy that you get for and once you have done this a couple of times it turns into a passionate stay, so every time that you experience pressure or grict, it triggers you to cat something.

Grapples keep you attached to convictions that you have about your life and yourself that prevent you from pushing ahead. You regularly compensate yourself with things that prevent you from

71

losing weight. When you're utilizing nourishment to reward or repay yourself, you are managing stays.

Although the grapples that I am alluding to around passionate eating are not healthy ones, they can likewise he utilized intentionally to get a specific outcome.

Enthusiastic eating doesn't happen because you are physically hungry. It occurs because something triggers a craving for nourishment. You are cither intuitively or deliberately covering a hidden, enthusiastic need.

The fear of eating can assume control over your life. It expends your musings, depleting you of your vitality and self-discipline, making you separate and gorge. This will create more fear and make matters more regrettable.

So how might you conquer your fear and different feelings around eating?

You can transform the majority of your feelings around eating into another more beneficial relationship

In all actuality, you have a soul. You should find it. It is that spot inside of you that is continually cherishing, forgiving and tranquil. It's a spot that speaks to your higher self.... the genuine you.... the sheltered, loved and entire you. When you find this, the resentment, dissatisfaction, and stress that you are feeling about your weight will vanish.

Things never appear to happen as fast as we might want them to...perhaps your body isn't changing as quickly as you need. This may demoralize you giving you further reason to indulge. Comprehend that your body is a gift, and afterward, you will begin to contemplate it.

Obesity and Eating Disorders

Eat delicious food. If you read this, you are one of the lucky people who have access to plenty of food. You can go to your closet or fridge and find something to cook. Otherwise, you can drive to the store or phone to go. Anyway, the point is there is a lot to do. The next point is to eat is a pleasure. It is an opportunity to involve our senses in something delicious. It also offers social opportunities having dinner with friends or chatting at the table with the family after a day off.

However, eating becomes a problem when we turn to it to deal with our emotions. You can feel happy, sad, stressed, worried, helpless, angry, excited ... They are all good excuses to cat. Instead of eating when you are hungry, let your feelings determine when you cat (and what, quite often). Suddenly you start using food to feel better about the events in your life. You have ended a relationship with your food that is much more complex than it should be.

What you should do is learn to use NO food to cope with everything that happens in your life. The ideal situation is to enjoy your food as it is and nothing else. Something delicious and nutritious that gives your body the energy you need to survive. You also need to be able to deal with things in your life in a way that doesn't involve food, but brings real change.

Emotional Eating

Emotional Eating - Don't let food control your life.

Most people ate at one time or another for emotional reasons. It can be the thought to turn when there is stress,

Eating to control emotions over a long period of time can have negative consequences. One of the biggest problems with using food to control emotions is that it can cause weight problems and there are many other problems associated with weight.

Emotional food is used to calm a number of emotions, such as: B. sadness, anger, frustration, loneliness or boredom, to name a few. Emotional hunger is different from physical hunger (the real reason to eat) and you are looking for food to meet emotional needs. We know that eating cannot ultimately satisfy an emotional need because it is supposed to satisfy physical hunger.

The starting point for emotional nutrition is to know whether you are getting involved. Honestly, many people do not know what they're doing and think they're just overeating. The foods that are chosen for emotional feeding are usually the ones you would consider comforting: rich in fats, salt, and sugar.

Here are some signs of emotional eating:

- Eat when you are not hungry.

- Eat when you experience feelings.

- Eat in isolation

- Eat and feel guilty later

- •.Overeating and not knowing why

- Eat to feel better

- Longing for food for no apparent reason and the thought that you cannot live without it

- Emotional feeding can increase because it tastes good at first and there are all positive thoughts about how much you want or need. The positive feelings (relief, calm) of emotional eating only last for a certain period of time (from one minute to hours), followed by a turning point at which you experience the following situations

- Feel guilty

- Shameful

- You feel upset because you overestimate.

- The feeling of a revival of the original feeling that triggered the attack.

- Be upset that you have gained or gained weight.

Your Relationship with Food

Take the time to think about your relationship with food. Has it changed over the years? Have there been any events that triggered the change, or do you remember that when you were a child you turned to eating at all in stressful times? Was it a change in circumstances? When couples move in together, women in particular are known to eat more than before and often as much as their partner.

You need to know your current eating habits before you can change them. Keep a close eye on what you eat and when you cat it for a week. Set when to use your emotions to determine when and what you cat. Are there certain emotions that attract you to cat? Note that you are in a specific mood when there are shifts in what you cat. Seek to be mindful of the amount you eat, t00 your goal is to focus on enjoying food in itself as a pleasure, not healing other wounds. It's no use feeling had about the food you cat, either. Instead, focus on how the food feels, the tastes and textures in your mouth. Most satisfaction comes when you cat something early on. So just enjoy the moment. Recognize you deserve to care for yourself. You deserve to get the best out of your body and you'll get some bonuses to look after. Food gives you the ability to live your life, allowing you to do anything you want. There is no need for emotional eating in a life so fun-filled!

If you know that all foods are all right in moderation then you're not going to end up overeating on your so-called forbidden' foods you resort to when you feel down.

If you have days, where you believe like food is the only way to go, excuse yourself when it happens. It's not the end of the planet and you failed not. Get on with your day then shrug your shoulders. Don't give yourself another cookie to try to get rid of the unpleasant sensations

If you want to, then go for it. Eating is a privilege and if you really like it you will eat it. But please enjoy it. Enjoy it for what it is food that gives your strength and your taste buds a pleasure. It won't stop your boss from being a psycho in charge, or settle your dispute with your wife. They need separate solutions

CHAPTER 14

CREATE A HEALTHIER RELATIONSHIP WITH FOOD EXERCISE

- Do you struggle to eat well nourishment?

- Do you attempt to imagine you appreciate eating soundly, however following two or three days, you truly miss your ordinary nourishments?

- Do you think that it's hard to eat well nourishment reliably?

If you genuinely need to create smart dieting propensities, at that point, this clear, standard hypnosis audio can support you. Also, to our "stop comfort eating" title, this will change your whole demeanor towards nourishment. Dissimilar to the stop comfort eating collection where a ton of the attention is likewise on creating mental quality and self-discipline to oppose urges. This collection truly centers around this side of things more - to help you develop good dieting propensities by re-wiring how you consider nourishment on a more profound subconscious level.

You will think about the negatives of eating an unfortunate eating routine.

Compared to seeing desserts, cheap foods, or just the greasy nutrition you like, you will think of the negative factors-weight gain, harmful health advice, and how low and low self-esteem you will feel after eating.

- You will likewise usually think about the positives of good dieting, how it will help you lose weight, improve your well-being, and how awesome and positive you will feel about yourself and how to defeat your solace eating inclinations! This specific change from negative to positive reasoning will profoundly affect your dietary patterns, and you will think that it's a lot simpler and considerably more characteristic to eat vigorously.

- You will turn out to be progressively predictable in your dietary patterns. You will stop "yo-yo-ing" between eating soundly, not all that strong, and pigging out. You will generally eat a significantly more adjusted and sounder eating routine, substantially more reliably.

- Finally, smart dieting will quit being a struggle for you as you build up the sort of attitude shared by the individuals who usually eat steadily without contemplating it. This last change in mentality and convictions will transform you, decrease your waistline, and change how you consider nourishment until the end of time.

What to expect

If you are new to hypnosis, at that point, you will locate this a fantastic encounter. You will turn out to be increasingly looser as you proceed to tune in. Reliant upon your learning style, you could conceivably recollect all aspects of the experience; you will anyway consistently stir feeling revived and lively.   Short term Over the short term, you will encounter genuine, substantial outcomes practically straight away. You will get yourself less powerless to enticements, and merely settling on better nourishment decisions naturally. You will feel significantly more positive about yourself and your capacity to remain "on track" and create enduring, positive, smart dieting propensities.   Long term After some time, the hypnotic recommendations will construct and make perpetual, enduring changes to your examples of reasoning and conviction sets related to yourself, abstaining from excessive food intake, and nourishment. You will steadily get one of those individuals who usually eat strongly. You won't fight or need to "be acceptable," you will generally eat a reasonable, sound eating regimen.

In light of this, you will wind up shedding pounds, getting more advantageous and more advantageous, and capitalizing on life!

Fussy eating habits: Can hypnotherapy help?

Getting kids to eat steadily can be testing, not to mention attempting to get them to demonstrate an eagerness to eat the soil products – especially when they are continually present to such a large number of low-quality nourishment options. Numerous parents of particular eaters are very acquainted with the catch-22 situation circumstance; they would prefer to see their kid eat garbage than releasing them hungry. Justifiable. In any case, is it accomplishing more damage than anything else over the long term? If the propensity proceeds for a delayed period, it might bring about the kid get- ting all the more requesting about the nourishments they eat – which may have a durable and harming impact on their association with nourishment. Yet, there are treatment alternatives accessible; hypnotherapy is one demonstrated technique for helping particular eaters change their association with food. We addressed the Hypnotherapy Directory part Penny Ling about how she moves toward hypnotherapy for customers with particular dietary patterns and how it can change their association with nourishment for good.

What Are The Typical Fundamental Issues of Fussy Eaters?

Most of the individuals who see me about particular eating issues are commonly youthful grown-ups in their 20s. They have built up the case by and large in adolescence and discover they can't change their dietary patterns. The explanation they have built up this issue differs, yet hidden problems come up repeatedly.

For in- stance:

- Something horrendous occurred, and they built up a profound dread or contempt of specific kinds of nourishment.

- Their folks had constrained weight control plans themselves.

I had a customer who, presently in her 50s, was fat and needed to lose weight. She had created particular eating as a kid when she went into the clinic matured 4 for an activity. Her eating regimen comprised of minced meat, potatoes, and peas in a wide range of structures – hamburger burgers and chips, cabin pie, mincemeat pie and potatoes, and so on Kids are typically attracted to better nourishments and regularly hate unpleasant food sources until their late adolescents. You likewise discover the appearance of nourishment will periodically be a piece of the issue, as well. All things being equal, our precursors gave special consideration to what they were eating, as new nourishments could slaughter you, so this sense is well and part of what makes us human. In any case, nourishment is frequently not the main problem.

How would you approach hypnotherapy for a fussy eater?

I utilize a blend of nourishing therapy and hypnotherapy for my particular eating customers.

They record in three segments:

1. What they at present eat.

2. What they might genuinely want to attempt.

3. What they will not eat.

Like this, we can deal with gradually bringing new nourishments into their eating routine. The hypnotherapy brings down their nervousness of attempting the new nourishments or scrambling any horrible encounters with nourishment, such as food contamination. I likewise show care, so come to dinner times they feel engaged and loose, not worried about what may be landing on the table. I also urge them to cook more; if you are setting up dinner, you comprehend what's in it.

What sort of results expected? To what extent does a treatment plan regularly last? The length of treatment relies particularly upon how upsetting the customers find attempting new nourishments. Some need some direction; others need their feelings of anxiety brought down first before attempting their eating plans. It shifts between four to 12 weeks, normally. It tends to be longer with youngsters, and regularly a parent likewise has the issue – along these lines, helping them is frequently the principal need. What exhortation would you provide for parents of particular eaters? First of all, try not to let the eating time become willful and scattered and right dieting conditions. Eat dinners as a family at the table, as kids see grown-ups eating a wide assortment of nourishments and frequently will need to attempt them themselves. Continuously offer the sound choice first and have a lot of foods grown from the ground to hand.

Try not to utilize treats as an insistence. "In case you're a decent young lady, you can have a few desserts" can set them on a terrible eating system forever – trust me, it's frequently been the issue with a ton of weight reduction customers of mine throughout the years. Try not to go into an "eat everything on your plate; there are starving kids in Africa" routine – this can prompt gorging.

CHAPTER 15

VIRTUAL AND ACTUAL GASTRIC BAND HYPNOSIS

Gastric Band Hypnosis Sessions

The person lies down, closes his eyes, and let's himself guide by the voice of the hypnotist. This voice will suggest to the brain that a surgeon is putting a ring on him that will shrink the stomach (by projecting it directly into the operating room) and make him record an intense feeling of satiety after a certain number of bites. The patient will then projects into a positive visualization of the result by seeing himself in a mirror with the silhouette he wishes to obtain. He will thus visualize his future with this new eating behavior in an enjoyable way, and a feeling of great satisfaction and self-realization will be deeply impressed. In addition to this session, psychological support work adds, always under hypnosis, to become aware of your body, manage compulsions, difficulty assimilating food, and the obstacles to this project's success. The aim is to encourage, maintain, and develop a deep motivation for lasting change. Regarding the number of sessions, 3 or 4 performed in the same week should be sufficient. They generally last 25 to 40 minutes (the longest being the first concerning the gastric band). Before starting, a first appointment fixes to know the eating habits, the psychological course, and the patient's exact expectations.

Some hypnotherapists sometimes ask for 2 to 3 more sessions, a few weeks after the method, incase the weight does not drop anymore, or the patient loses his motivation.

The Protocol of the Virtual Gastric Band

The protocol establishes over five sessions spaced 2 to 3 weeks apart:

- **First Nutrition session:** it highlights the physiological obstacles to weight loss. This session is essential.

- **First Hypnosis session:** a complete assessment of eating habits, goals, and emotional barriers to weight loss; this session makes it possible to define the priority axes of work and to adapt the management. A first hypnosis session sets up to prepare the patient to welcome the changes to come.

- **Second session:** this hypnosis session will allow you to work on eating behavior and compulsions management.

- **Third session:** this session, depending on the first results obtained, will be reserved for installing the virtual gastric band; it will, therefore, provide the feeling of reduced stomach.

- **Fourth session:** under hypnosis, the ring adjusts, and the work on eating behavior consolidated. This session strengthens your image and your self- confidence. It will also anchor the person you want to become permanent to make the results lasting.

The Principles of the Virtual or Hypnotic Gastric Band

A virtual gastric ring's installation reproduces your unconscious effects similar to surgical intervention without undergoing the side effects (fatigue, narcosis, and trauma). Your therapist will use your mental power to convince you that you have had a gastric banding with your collaboration. The virtual gastric band is a reliable and durable method since it eliminates frustration and restriction, making it possible to apprehend one's diet under a new eye, facilitating a qualitative diet being binding. Your therapist will be able to guide you to choose the type of hypnosis that best suits your needs, whether the problem is from the amount of intake, from the fuzzy feeling of hunger, from compulsive eating, psychological dependence on food, or emotional eating.

Your hypnotherapist will also guide you in more in-depth work, help you visualize your thinness, and regain your confidence in your ability to lose weight and maintain results.

Weight Loss and Virtual Gastric Band

Having a virtual gastric band can work with everyone, as long as they want to volunteer. It will create a feeling of narrowing the stomach and reprogram the unconscious's good physiological messages, often disturbed by many diets, stress, and repeated sleep disturbances. It is a reprogramming of the brain so that it can accept a new eating behavior. Thus, the person will learn to manage all his emotions using his mind and no longer by mouth. It is clear that this method is simple, without any danger or side effect, and therefore it is not subject to any contraindication.

The Virtual Gastric Band, a Tool to Control Your Weight

Millions of people are considered obese, a trend affecting all ages, which should further intensify in the coming years. Our way of life often favors these problems (inadequate diet, sedentary lifestyle). In addition to an increased risk of disease, obesity can lead to psychological distress, with some individuals feeling excluded from society. There has been an alternative to surgery, called virtual gastroplasty. It takes place under hypnosis and aims to relearn the brain to eat correctly. The gastric band under hypnosis does not involve any risk for the patient, who could seek a loss of weight that is certainly less spectacular, but more durable. The goal is to benefit from slimming's long-term benefits, including increased energy, less pain, and better self-image. During the sessions, the professional will suggest several avenues and elements, which will create strong motivational levers. This work will be vital to achieving your personal goals by solving deep-seated problems. It is by using the mental potential that we earn a real change. Hypnosis indeed uses to modify the perception that a person has on a particular thing: if, for example, the sweet aspect obsesses you, we will find together ways so that this flavor becomes repulsive in your eyes or loses its interest. With the virtual gastric band, the individual feels that there is something in his stomach that can bring him a satiety signal.

Sessions Developed to Achieve Your Goals

In practice, losing weight with a virtual gastric band simply consists of a series of personalized sessions, where the therapist places a gastric band with the particularity of being virtual. The goal is to influence and rectify the signal sent from the stomach to the brain. The support requires several sessions; it will not be possible to lose weight in a single visit. After that, you will quickly feel full when you ingest a small amount of food, in the same way as if you had benefited from a gastroplasty. There is no hunger, so there is no frustration due to deprivation, which maximizes the chances of lasting success, unlike diets. Following these conditioning sessions, the patient will be plunged into a hypnotic state, resembling for him a moment of relaxation. A series of mental images and suggestions will then be transmitted to him, all very simple to follow. This virtual gastric ring hypnosis will allow you to feel the decrease in stomach size. After that, additional sessions schedule if necessary, make certain adjustments, take into account emotional difficulties, or take stock of developments.

Controlling the Notions of Hunger and Satiety: The Advantages of Hypnosis

In summary, the virtual gastric band's establishment allows you to lose weight without massive efforts, only by setting your brain so that eating better and less be- comes obvious. The promises of this type of virtual gastric band hypnosis are available to obese people who don't want surgery, or those who just want to lose some weight. Surgical gastroplasty disadvantages are numerous: high cost, hospitalization, postoperative complications, and frequent side effects, not to mention that lifestyle habits brutally disrupt the operation. The virtual gastric band pose offers an entirely different approach: much more affordable, it does not involve the risk of anesthesia, pain, medical treatment, or side effects. Natural and safe, this program requires only a few appointments of about an hour and a half and will be easily adjustable on a case-by-case basis.

What is the Virtual Gastric Band Technique?

The method consists of placing a ring to lose weight by practicing a reduction in the stomach, but virtually without any real operation. A well-known British hypnotherapist developed this technology. Combining conscious hypnosis with neuro language programming (NLP) will help to adopt different eating habits. The recipient will, therefore, learn to feel full by taking smaller amounts of food. The surgical intervention of placement of the gastric band is, therefore, done only by visualization. And it is practiced in a comfortable setting by providing lasting weight loss, especially since it accompanies psychological care.

What Does Virtual Stomach Reduction Consist Of?

It includes clinical therapeutic hypnosis and losing weight and losing weight durably without a restrictive diet or surgical intervention. Your conscience makes you differentiate between a hypnosis session and surgical intervention, anesthesia, operational risks, and healing. This operation forces the patient to limit the amount of food he can eat, and it reserves for people with morbid obesity. As for your unconscious, it does not make the difference between a virtual or surgical gastroplasty. It is a pure and straightforward reduction in the stomach; therefore, it decreases your ingest food ability. And in this, your unconscious is right because after installing the virtual gastric band, it is as if you had benefited from a gastroplasty. Your body will react in the same way as if you had undergone surgery and will therefore request food in sufficient quantity to meet your need- s. You can eat what you want, but as the amounts will be appropriate to your needs, you will quickly feel full without deprivation or feeling of hunger.

CHAPTER 16

GASTRIC BAND HYPNOSIS PHASES

1. Hypnotizing Words For Gastric Band Placement

I will your guide on this mental journey, as we put a mental and emotional gastric band around your stomach, whose primary purpose is to permit you to feel a good fullness as soon as you eat precisely as much eat as you need. Get into a comfortable sitting position, preferably your favorite spot, so that you can remain undisturbed for the entire period of this magical procedure. The more you relax, the more the gastric band becomes more powerful and productive over your life. Take a big deep breath in - to relax and exhale tension and worry as you softly close your eye. Begin to feel your body already slowing down, take another breath at your pace, and let it go with a sigh. This moment is for you to practice a new lifestyle of being full at the perfect time for you. Now, say to yourself with conviction, overeating is impossible for me, and breath into the truth of these words, breathe them out into reality, creating a smaller stomach already.

Cool down, relax, breathe, and use the power of your imagination to visualize a beautiful beach with white sand reflecting in the sunlight, almost looking like snow. You will see the water fade to a deep blue as the ocean get deeper. Look down into the sand where you stand and notice sand grains, all in different colors and textures. Suddenly, something catches your eye, half-buried in the sand, it is your favorite color, so you get closer. Yes, go ahead and walk closer you will see a small thick band, about the size of your fist. Can you see it? Yes, you have seen it. And it's the most definitive version of your favorite color. The brightness of this band brings you strange excitement, inner happiness, and palpable joy. This curious round band flashing your most beloved color choice is called a GASTRIC BAND. It means to be placed around the top of your stomach organ, therefore reducing your stomach's capacity. In order words, it makes your stomach smaller, giving you the feeling of fullness when you've had enough to eat. This kind of band exists in the medical world. (However, during this relaxing process, by placing a band aid on your stomach, you can use the power of your creative thinking to achieve the same result.)

Now you are walking along this beach carrying your gastric band, feel it in your hand, notice the texture, the weight, and the thickness. Feel your feet in the sand, allow those steps to relax you more and more, and see the paltry surface and space under your feet. Let it deeply soothe you even while you feel the ocean breeze and smell the salty air, all along this beach. As you walk, you get a little tired from your long walk. Then a reclining chair has appeared just for you, facing the ocean. So, you have to sit and recline back. Remember, you still have your gastric band in your hand. By now, you are familiar with its shape and size; it has something like a small bolt that can be tightened and loosen. Relax

93

back in the chair and look at the endless waves of water before you; notice the ocean meeting with the sky, the clouds are streaming along ever so slowly on a bright blue backtrack. No one is around you; it's peaceful and relaxing; it's gorgeous. Feel the shining sun on your skin, kissing you with nutrients. Notice the warm sand under your feet; it is soft and soothing. Allow your breath to become a little bit deeper and more massive. Listen to the coming sound of the air coming in and out. It is similar to the sound of a wave crashing on a surf. Focus intently on the waves' relaxing and coming sound, gaze out upon the ocean in front of you, see the crystal-clear waters, ripening, and brewing and reflecting the rays of light, making the surface of the water tensed. If your mind starts wandering and you see some negativity or doubt about weight loss, show up, breathe into it. Let the wave come and take that thought back out to the oceans past the hole. Exhale, take a deep breath, and feel that you and the waves are the same. Breathe out a long breath out, feel the vibes of your body, and antagonism about your weight streak away, dissolving, getting less diverting in your psyche. Re- hash this excellent procedure of giving up self-question, full breath in, into the waves, full breath out, feel the hints of your negative self-talk start to wash away. Release everything and last time, benefit as much as possible from it, full breath in, into the waves, let them remember every one of your considerations. Your cynicism and stresses over ever eating and take a long full breath out, feel them smashing and vanishing, leaving for eternity.

2. Hypnotizing Words for Gastric Band Tightening

Welcome to this relaxing meditation that will guide you to a pristine lake surrounded by mountains so that you can tighten your gastric band, making for an even smaller stomach that fills up quickly. Get into a decent sitting position, some- place that you can completely give up and would not be upset by the encompassing scene. As you get into an excellent condition of unwinding and starting to envision that you are fixing this gastric band, you will discover that weight reduction gets more straightforward and more uncomplicated always. Start to inhale profoundly, permitting your body to ultimately grow and breathe out the entirety of your worry in one profound inhale out. Take another breath, and then exhale, closing the eyes delicately. Notice how you can feel your body settling down and getting considerably progressively loose as we go on. Relinquish any current concerns or commitments; appreciate this time by and by for yourself. Now say to yourself these words, "I eat only as much food as I need. I require less food to make me fill full." Breathing in, allowing these words to become authentic on every level of your awareness. Breathe out any doubt and breathe in the truth that you are capable of eating just the right amount to have the perfect shape, size, and overall wellness. Calm, relax entirely at ease, allow my voice to soothe you, every word I speak, let your body slow down, just a little bit more. Activate your imagination by bringing in into your mind eye the sight of a magnificent lake surrounded by mountains. The sky is a crystal-clear blue doubled with the occasional clouds; the sun is brightly shining all around you, the waters of this lake are crystal clear and reflect the blueness of the sky, the water almost acts as a mirror for the mountain range. Become aware of your stomach and how it's a little bit smaller from an excellent session on the beach when you first find your gastric band. Your gut is comfortable and happy about its new size, ready to become even smaller. As you walk towards this beautiful lake, you will notice the soil under your feet; it is smooth and supportive below. You get to the lake's edge and deep our toes in the cold and freshwater. Only your feet immerse, your entire body is getting too relaxed by the waters of the mystical lake. You will notice besides you that there is a small red canoe waiting for you. Get on this canoe, and it picks up its beautiful hand curve oar; this oar represents your ability to tighten your gastric band. Deep the oar in the water, all the way to the shallow bottom of the lake, push off the shore. You will see that this simple movement tightens your gastric band a little more in millimeter. Now, start paddling into the lake and admire the surrounding scenery, hearing water splashing on both sides of the boat; every time you immerse them in the water so that the ship can easily transport you, it will tighten your stomach—little by little. The weather is perfect; beautiful birds are flying overhead, tripping a melody for you. It is relatively too late for sensation, almost as if you are walking out of the gym and building muscle, losing ligaments and activating healthy blood flow, and you are merely rolling a boat in your mind. Stop moving now and just let the canoe glide through the water on its own. Please pay attention to the beautiful mountains on all sides, because they can protect the lake from bad weather, just as they can protect you from self-doubt, you can only meet your needs with every meal and every meal every day. Rest of life

And this choice is critical for you because you care about your health, you are passionate about feeling good and moving your body freely with ease and strength. Envision that you can see this excellent gastric band around the highest point of your stomach, delicately pressing it, making for the need for less food in other to make you full. The band is still your favorite color, shiny, and it feels like a big hug from the band to your belly, just like the hug you get from your famous grand-parents, uncles, or anyone you know. To comfort you, support you, and let you know that this band is here because you want it to exist.

3. Hypnotizing Words for Gastric Band Removal

Welcome to this relaxing session to remove your gastric band. So far, you have placed this band around your stomach by walking on a relaxing beach and then tightening this band while rowing your canoe on a crystal-clear lake. Today, we will now visit an ancient Japanese castle to remove this band and discard it during a beautiful ceremony. It is your final step in your gastric band experience. Take a nice deep breath in, and as you breathe out, close your eyes. Relax your body; it sinks into the chair or bed, is soft and robust underneath it, and moves in and out. Become aware of your abdomen and how much slimmer it is each day, little by little, because you eat less food. You fill up quickly; hunger is a thing of the past. You know when you have to eat, however, it doesn't expend your day or your night, and you simply eat when you have to and don't eat when you don't have to, as raw as that. Activate your creative mind once again; imagine that you are standing in a beautiful filled with tall grass blowing in the wind. The floors and the golden drums around the doors and windows still keep the building in good condition.

CHAPTER 17

GBH 2.0 (3 STEP) PART ONE

During this session, your body will gradually learn to respond to suggestions in a way that reduces your appetite. Slowly, you will start to feel fuller after eating smaller amounts of food, similar to the gastric band surgery. As you visualize going through the procedure, and the more you repeat this process, the better your body responds to the suggestions. You will start to feel like your stomach has, indeed, reduced, and fewer calories are enough to satisfy your cravings than before. With each repetition, the procedure will start to look more realistic, and you will feel a more substantial, more noticeable effect. First, let's briefly address diets and address some of the reasons why you might have failed to lose weight in the past. Failing with diets wasn't your fault, and it doesn't speak badly about your personality. Gently release any guilt and shame associated with the fact that, in the past, you might have tried to maintain a steady diet but failed at it. Most diets are temporary and are hard to sustain in the long run. It's not you who is the problem. The problem you faced with dieting had to do with the fact that overly restrictive diets aren't effective. They deprive not only foods and nutrients, but also pleasure and fulfillment needed for long-term success. With this hypnosis, you will virtually commit to yourself to change your habits and the way of eating. As you subconsciously receive the virtual gastric band, you will gradually, through suggestions, gain the confidence and discipline needed to establish healthy eating habits. These habits will reflect on the way you eat, go through your day, and exercise. Over time, the beneficial changes will build up to support your long-term, healthy weight loss and improve your physical health. First, let's briefly discuss your weight loss experiences, eating patterns, and your general health and relationship with food. Mimicking the gastric band surgery will help you create an authentic virtual experience, incorporating imagery, sounds, and smells you'd feel while undergoing this operation. In a deep hypnotic state, you will go through the procedure. This hypnosis will take you to step by step through the process of this surgery.

Part Two

Welcome to your gastric band hypnosis. In this hypnosis, you will receive a virtual gastric band. This way, you will lose weight healthily and beneficially for your body and mind. The suggestions you'll receive are healthful, helpful, and positive, and won't harm you in any way. Whenever you want to, you can reinforce these suggestions by repeating this hypnosis. First, let's relax to open your mind to positive suggestions. Now, you'll start receiving offers to be in a state of relaxation, so that you can virtually and mentally in- stall the hypnotic gastric band. Sit down and begin to relax. Focus on my voice. As you listen to my voice, you're becoming more and more relaxed. Keep relaxing, shrugging, and dropping your shoulders until they're free of any pressure. Look around you, and inwards, into your body, to detect any tightness or discomfort. If you see tension, relax the part of your body that feels tight. Relax any places in your body that feel uncomfortable. Now, I will start counting from ten to one. When I finish counting, you will feel entirely relaxed in every part of your body.

Each piece of your body will become fully relaxed.

- Ten. Breathe in, pause, and let the breath out. Breathe deeply, directing the breath into your stomach.

- Nine. Pause for a second time, and let the breath out.

- Eight. Breathe in for the third time, hold, and breathe out. Now, you are feeling much, much better.

- Seven. You are breathing relaxed, breathing tension, and discomfort. Your mind becomes calm and quiet with each breath.

- Six. You are more and more calm and quiet. Everything around you is serene, warm, and safe. You hear only the sounds of this hypnosis—all chores, worries, and stress fade into the distance.

- Five. Breathe in relaxation, and breathe out tiredness. With each exhale, you're sinking deeper into relaxation. Deeper and deeper, until you feel weightless and completely safe.

- Four. Relaxation washes over your face, jaw, and your lips.

Your neck is softer, shoulders relaxed. Relaxation spreads through your body, your shoulders, back, chest, and stomach. You are softening your thighs, calves, and feet. You are soft, safe, and relaxed. You are diving deeper and deeper into relaxation, as you breathe deeply in and out. Your hands are resting beside you, completely relaxed. There's no need to move; you are simply calm and relaxed. There's nothing else to do but to sink further into relaxation. Your body is opening up, loosening, softening, and breathing into relaxation.

As you exhale, your body sinks further into your chair. Letting go feels beautiful. You are drifting and floating into heavy relaxation. Three, your legs are becoming more massive, and you're focusing on your feet as they become calm and loose.

- At two, all of your body is relaxed. Remember, you're in control.

- One. You are letting go of everything but the sense of relaxation.

You are completely comfortable, relaxed, and at ease. You are sitting comfortably; your mind is open. You are receptive to my suggestions. Your mind and body are deeply connected. Open your mind now. Accept and allow positive, healthy ideas into your mind to boost your resources and strengths. Your mind is clear and open. You look forward to the change waiting to happen. You are calm and excited. The quality of life and vitality will improve this positive change. You are thrilled and hope to bring positive changes. You are entering a hospital corridor. You're hearing sounds of visitors and looking at medical staff. The smells of clean, hygiene products, and disinfectants you can feel. Everything is fresh and clean. You are safe and about to experience a change in your attitude towards food. You are starting a transition to uplift your body and mind. You are lying in a hospital bed. A nurse is there beside you, just to care for you. She is calm and encouraging. The nurse is smiling at you. You trust and like her, so you smile back at her. She touches your hand, and you feel happy and comforted. Turn around, and notice the bright lights in the room. You surround by bright white and blue lights. These lights make you feel sleepy and tired. Your eyes feel heavy, and your breath is light and even. There are several people there, and you feel like you're drifting deeper and deeper into nesthesia. Your stomach feels a sense of excitement that grows within you. Nothing matters but this safety and excitement about a fresh start. You are relaxed in this room, surrounded by warm blue lights. Feel the softness of the hospital bed. Focus on feeling relaxed and comfortable as a soft bed supports your back. The nurse points a bright light at you, and you can only see the shadows of medical staff walking around. Something cold touches your stomach, and something inside begins to change. You are drifting away and starting to observe yourself on the bed. You see yourself surrounded by doctors, nurses, and instruments. Now, a doctor makes a small incision into your stomach, a tiny one. They fit the band inside. Just like that, the process is quickly over. Now, you see the staff walking away. Everyone is relaxed and happy, and so are you. The job finishes, such little time was enough. Now, you are getting better and better. Now, you choose to eat sensibly and to have only the right foods. These foods heal your body and mind. You only desire healthy meals that are nutritious, abundant in fruits and vegetables. Foods feel lovely as you chew and swallow. They are healthy, tasty, satiating. You only desire healthy, lean, nourishing foods in the perfect amounts. Your stomach feels light and comfortable. Your subconscious and conscious mind choose this. You feel at ease. You feel well, energized, and hydrated. You're noticing how your stomach feels full as you finish the right amount. You no longer need to eat after your stomach feels full. You have now developed healthy habits, a healthy outlook on food and diet. You look forward to health and listen to your body. Everything should be so. Eat when you are hungry. You feel the difference between sadness and hunger, fear and desire, boredom, and need. When you feel these emotions, you inhale and exhale deeply. You no longer cover them up with food. As you're relaxing, your mind relaxes softly. You are changing as you breathe. With every breath, you become stronger and more competent, resourceful. You are sure of yourself. You think of yourself in different ways. You know and believe that you can change your habits for the better. The way you think and feel affects how you act. You're choosing to eat correctly. You're choosing to eat with confidence and awareness, and when you're starving. Changes happen within weeks, as you learn to listen to your body and mind. It is the role of hyno band. You have more control, and you feel right. Eat right, a flat abdomen, calm energy, you don't want to overeat. After a couple of weeks, you feel more energy. Clearly and calmly, you see new possibilities and opportunities. You smile with pride in your achievement. You're trying on new clothes and fit in them easily. You're more excited, and you have more energy. You enjoy moving and exercising. You want healthy foods, and the softness and flavor of protein, fruits, and vegetables. You become healthier and slimmer. Your posture is tall, head held high. Everything is in its place. You are healthy and happy.

After the Hypnosis

After you go through the gastric band hypnosis process, you will gradually start craving more healthy foods. The subconscious suggestions you received will train your brain to send the message of feeling full after eating less food. If you're overeating, you will start to recognize being physically robust. In the past, this could have been difficult. With hypnosis, you'll start noticing the difference be- tween being hungry and being full. You will begin to notice small, barely noticeable physical sensations that appear as you get hungry, and you'll start detecting how you feel when you start feeling full. It will set the basis for you to start developing healthy eating habits. Moreover, the hypnosis will feel safe, relaxing, and pleasant, helping you build a calmer approach to reviewing intrinsic issues surrounding food, your body, and weight. With the gastric band hypnosis, you'll reap all the benefits of the experience, but without the physical pains of recovery. You won't experience any nausea, acid reflux, or vomiting. Physical symptoms of the surgery won't manifest, as the experience is entirely psychological. Ultimately, whether or not the gastric band hypnosis will work for you depends on many factors. You might notice behavioral changes and changes in sensations soon after your first session, or it could take multiple sessions before you see any changes. Either way, you should be patient and allow the changes to manifest in a way that's natural to you and your mind.

CHAPTER 18

USING HYPNOSIS TO CONTROL FOOD PORTIONS

If you want to reduce your weight, the first thing you have to think about is how to minimize your food consumption. You know that your value has risen because you have eaten more food than you need, and it is urgent to fix the issue. Therefore, the most straightforward answer is to minimize the amount of food you eat, and your weight will disappear for good. That's real, but there's a catch. You can feel hungry by merely reducing your food intake. This feeling of hunger is more than tolerable for most people, and they tend to let their eating plan fall. As a consequence, they cannot lose weight. Nevertheless, there are ways you can get back into shape without ever feeling hungry. The first thing you have to do is know the types of food you consume. You will most likely learn that many of your everyday foods contain very high calories. It is these kinds of foods that you have to try to stop. You should exclude ready meals and snacks from your diet because they contain almost always significant quantities of calories. Fizzy foods, beer, and colas all have a lot of sugar and have to omit from your diet. Dairy products usually contain plenty of fat, and you should select the low-fat calorie alternative, if available, wherever possible. You should also start consuming more natural suppressants of hunger every day. Most of the green leafy vegetables have very few calories and a high nutrient content, which will make you feel quicker. You should strive to include as many green leafy vegetables as possible in your meals. Healthy salads are also a great way to help you lose weight. Your brain usually takes about 20 minutes to acquire gastric signals, indicating that it has enough food. Eating a small salad dish as a starter before your main meal will make it easier to cut portion sizes drastically. You can't cover your salad in any way since they all contain large quantities of calories, even the slimmer versions. If you can't enjoy a salad without some sort of dressing, but a little beside the plate to check how much you eat. Try eating more fish in your diet. In omega-3, salmon, herring, and tuna are all strong. It helps to increase your body's leptin, which helps control your desire to eat. Fresh fruit like apples is perfect for weight loss. Apples require a lot of chewing as they also contain a lot of pectin's and soluble fiber, which boosts your energy. No one will go for appetite suppressant diet pills if they know how easy it is to safely control calorie intake by almost 50 percent and lose weight. If you know this trick, you no longer need to waste money on a low-calorie diet, unhealthy food packets, and expensive appetite suppressants. Clear guidelines or strategies for effective dieting: Drink two cups of water between meals. Break into medium pieces and scatter on the cucumber, tomatoes, carrots, beetroot and onion, black pepper powder, and lemon juice (depending on your taste). Eat at least 15 pieces of cut vegetables before each meal (numbers matter, you eat more, you feel half full). Keep two fruits or two fresh apples with you while eating (for psychological effect!). You want to maintain room in the stomach and eat less when you look at them. Is it not simple? You're not going to get sick with such meals. You do not expect to sacrifice any kind of food to lose weight. By using this strategy alone, you will lose almost 8 pounds in a month. Besides lowering your calorie consumption by 50%, you can achieve a weight loss of 10-12 pounds in a month if you follow a few more straight- forward guidelines. Take 3 to 5 drops of citrus juice early in the morning.

Drink at least one to two glasses of water 4-6 times a day. Exercise for 30 minutes to one hour every day (the heartbeat rate should be higher than usual). Drink two glasses of water before going to bed. You don't have to spend even a penny on weight loss pills and plans in the fu- ture if you obey the above diet strategies and regulations. Normal suppression of appetite and a little workout to improve your metabolism will help to lose weight safely. Often ignored are the risks associated with appetite suppressants: elevated blood pressure & heart rate, restlessness, nervousness, insomnia, and dry mouth. People aware of the dangers seek natural ways to thwart their hunger pangs. The famous natural advice is to drink more water and increase fiber intake. For most people, this doesn't do the job. But instead of going along with the "more water + fiber" slogan, let's discuss a few hormones that determine whether or not we feel hungry or satiated and fulfilled for some hours. Ideally, we want to eat a meal and stay energized for some hours. We need to keep our insulin on the low side. One simple way we can do this is by reducing our sugars / starchy carb intake and combining our meals with plenty of healthy fats and quality proteins. The added fat, in particular, will protect against potential blood sugar crashes. Following a collision, people tend to overeat and sometimes pick the wrong foods. It is something we want to stop. GLUCAGON is the counter-hormone to insulin. It allows us to maintain the equilibrium of blood sugar and retain energy between meals. We inhibit the release of glucagon when we consume a meal that is primarily sugar or carb. Therefore, you are likely to feel happy longer than snacking on a big apple if you eat half of the apple with some macadamia nuts. PEPTIDE YY (PYY) is a hormone frequently neglected for the control of appetite. It ought not to be! One of our hormones tells us when to avoid eating when we are satiety. Carbohydrate does not emit a lot of PYY while protein and fat are re- leased. This is why overcrowding a bag of chips is so easy. PYY doesn't tell us to stop! That is also why merely growing the intake of fibers (usually carbohydrate) to sus- tain appetite may not work for all.—fiber can make you feel "full" somehow, bloat- ed. But you still won't feel relaxed for many hours. Adequate PROTEIN + QUALITY PROTEIN = APPETITE MANAGEMENT

Having understood how insulin, glucagon, and PYY play a role in hunger sig- nals, you may already have concluded that foods that prioritize healthy fats and quality protein would keep you more satisfied and energized than meals with car- bohydrates. For example, a bagel and juice breakfast will: —increase the amount of your insulin —make you hungry a few hours from the inhibited release of glucagon and minimal out of PYY. An omelet/spinach and other vegetable breakfast and maybe a little bit of cheese: —keep insulin on the low side —Keep you happy for many hours because a lot of glucagon and PYY is re-leased.

Tips For Control Appetite Naturally

1. Start the day with protein- and fat-rich foods such as chopped eggs with veg- etables or dinner leftovers the night before.

2. Instead of making a starchy, carb-centered food such as a sandwich and pasta cup, choose to dress extra virgin olive oil, herbs, and apple cider vinegar as a giant salad with quality meat/fish healthy fats from avocado, chives, or homemade salads.

3. Keep something handy like deviled eggs, sliced avocados, a handful of macadamia noodles, jerky, or a Tanka bar for a midday snack. Smart snacks like this help to discourage overeating.

4. Choose protein for dinners, such as meat/fish cooked with healthy fat and veggies.

5. You can catch a spoonful of coconut cream or cocoon oil in a time rush be- fore your meal.

6. DO NOT EAT FAT! Fat is your companion when it comes to managing your appetite. It is the sup- pressive hunger of mother nature. If you're thinking about fat calories – don't be. Portion sizes begin to decrease when hunger signals are fully operational.

CHAPTER 19

MEDITATIONS

Why Frustration Killing Your Weight Loss, How To Avoid Frustration With Meditation Hypnosis And Affirmations Phrases With 1 Hour Guided Exercise

When it comes to rapid weight loss, meditation is one technique that acts like secret weapons. Studies conducted on meditation and mindfulness have shown that these exercises link to weight loss. They not only boost an individual's awareness but also banish belly fat and lower stress levels. Having an attentive mind can help you avoid binge or emotional eating.

What is Meditation?

Meditation refers to the practice of clearing your mind daily so you can have calm and peaceful thinking. Most people only took a few minutes to meditate in a day, while others take up to half an hour.   Meditation must not be a difficult technique. If you are a beginner, take only five minutes when you wake up to clear your mind before you start your day. You just need to close your eyes and focus your mind on your goals as you breathe in and out. As you live, don't let your mind wander, and if this happens, simply guide

it back without making any judgment.

What is the Connection between Meditation and Weight Loss?

Meditation is known to be a useful tool for weight loss. It aligns the unconscious mind with the conscious mind to facilitate changes that we want to make in our behaviors. Such modifications your unconscious mind must become engaged in the change process because of weight-gaining, poor habits such as emotional eating cultivation. Through meditation, you will be able to become more aware of your surroundings and will be able to overcome your unhealthy habits. But there is even a more immediate effect of mediation. It can reduce the level of stress hormones in the body. Hormones like cortisol give the body signal to store more calories. If you have high cortisol levels moving through your system, it will be challenging to cut down weight even if you are eating healthy foods. Most of us stress most cases, but it takes only 25 minutes of meditation three times to re- duce stress. In 2016, a study conducted by Texas Tech University found that increased relaxation, attention, body-mind awareness, calmness, and brain activity result from just a few meditation sessions. The researchers found that the brain is most affected by reflection, which means that with a few minutes of meditation, you will be able to pass by that ice cream when feeling stressed.

How to Start Meditating for Weight Loss

Even without training, anyone who has a body and mind can practice meditation. For most of us, the most challenging aspect of meditation is getting time. You can start with as little as 8 to 10 minutes a day. Ensure that you can access a quiet place for meditation. You may even practice your mediation while in the shower. Once you are in a place of silence, take a comfortable position. You can either lie down or sit in a situation that makes you feel at ease. Start meditating by putting your focus on your breath. Watch the way your stomach or chest rises and falls. Feel the air that you breathe in and out of your mouth. Listen keenly to the sounds around you. It should do for 2 or 3 minutes until you begin feeling relaxed.

Then, do the following steps:

- Take in a deep breath, and hold for a few seconds

- Slowly breathe out, and repeat the process

- Breathe in a natural manner

- Observe how your breath enters your nostrils, influence your chest's movement, and move your stomach.

- Continue focusing on the way you breathe in and out for about 8 to 10 minutes

- Your mind may begin to wonder, which a regular

occurrence is. Just acknowledge this and return your attention to the process

- As you wrap up, reflect on your thoughts, and acknowledge how you can quickly bring your mind together

Benefits of Meditation on Weight Loss

Below are the incredible ways that meditation can help you achieve daily weight loss: Meditation reduces stress

With permanent roles in life, including work, children, and home activities, it is not surprising that you may be overwhelmed, which may contribute to increased stress. As a result, the hormone causes weight gain. Studies have revealed that meditation activates a relaxation response, regulating the nervous system and, in turn, lowering the cortisol levels. With a few minutes of deep breathing and conscious relaxation, you will be able to obtain the cortisol-lowering benefits as well as your overall stress levels. Meditation promotes a focus on intention often, meditation techniques involve focusing on specific goals or concepts. Meditating on cutting down weight streams your energy, thoughts, and intentions to a particular purpose. The outspoken meaning will stay with you for a long while, enabling you to achieve your weight loss goal both consciously and subconsciously, and dodging all possible distractions. With meditation, you will learn conscious eating

With daily meditation, you will be able to boost your levels of mindfulness and awareness. It can allow you to live in the moment and always focus on what you are doing in the present. The meditation process can help you gain an increased sense of awareness of actions and thoughts, thus allowing you to think twice be- fore taking action. Rather than enabling your cravings to take over you, you will develop the power of controlling your mind, thus handling your desires with greater intention and awareness. When you are ready to eat, your attention will make it easier to recognize the textures and flavors of the food you are eating, instead of taking them for granted. Meditation stabilizes mood hormones

Daily stressors and activities can affect how your system usually operates and may throw your hormones out of normal functioning. Apart from keeping your cortisol and adrenaline levels regulated, meditation goes further than this. The relaxation technique releases both oxytocin and serotonin hormones, which boost your moods and ensure your hormones remain stable. Meditation regulates sleep   Lack of sleep may hinder your weight loss progress. You see, by having a deep sleep, your cortisol levels will rise, which in turn will sabotage your progress in losing weight. With meditation, you will be able to balance the circadian rhythms that promote quality sleep. Meditation increases the levels of melatonin, a hormone that also determines and controls when you sleep.

How to Make Sure that Meditation Works for You

If you want to include meditation in your rapid weight loss hypnosis, you must make it simple. Meditation should help you recover from any stressful event, not become a source of it. That is why you need to consider the three easy ways high- lighted below, which you can incorporate in your daily mediation.

Make an Affirmation That Can Help You Lose Weight

A mantra refers to a phrase that one repeats to focus their mind on mediation and bring them to the relaxation state. A mantra can give help you identify something to focus on as you meditate. Although it is beneficial to many people, a mantra is not a must in meditation. You don't need to force yourself to use one if you don't find it helpful or if it does not make you feel natural. However, if you choose to use one, you need to repeat it as you inhale and when you exhale. Some of the common mantras used include "I am at peace with myself," "I am loved," or "I can do this."

Follow Your Breath to Avoid Stress

As you meditate, try to count your inhales four ties and exhales eight times. Remember that meditation is a process to reduce stress; if these counts do not feel natural, you should deviate from them. Every time you meditate, always try to increase the number of exhaling and inhaling counts. Do not feel stressed if it takes longer to reach eight counts. Just keep in mind that lengthening the exhale will significantly affect your health as you will calm down.

Consider a Guided Meditation

If you are not able to practice meditation alone, you should consider a guided process. It includes websites, phone apps, podcasts, and recordings that can help you connect with experts who show you how to meditate.

How to Create a Meditation Space at Home

You may find it easier to practice meditation daily to motivate your weight loss process. Creating and incorporating meditation accessories and organizing the right space might help you throughout the practice. Some of the equipment to get started, including:

Essential Oil Diffuser

Aromatherapy is considered a useful calming tool for the body, which is very helpful during meditation. An essential oil diffuser can help you create a relaxing environment to reap the essential oils' benefits. Additionally, the diffuser always shuts off when the water runs out; thus, you can meditate as long as you like.

Bluetooth Earbud Headphones

Don't have enough space to practice your meditation? You may consider wireless headphones, which you can to wherever you go. The headphones can sync up with Android and iPhones devices, which you can use to listen to your best-guided mediation without bothering those close to you.

A Meditation Filled Cotton Pillow Cushion

A meditation cushion can give you comfort to find a point of relaxation. The pillow will relieve you from stress, especially after having a prolonged sitting period. It has the perfect density and height to sit through for hours of meditation practice.

How To Heal Your Body?

What does your body tell you in your own life of the need to heal the wound? Every day, the body sends out signals which let you know how safe it is in general. Aches and pains are usually a warning somewhere deep inside that something are wrong. Some of the origins are a little more obvious than others. You need to spend some time listening to the tips about the overall health of your body.

Positive Thought

Nearly every religion in the world states that positive thinking plays a significant role in healing. When you have to heal the body, it is good to spend a little time thinking each day positively. You may just find that in this age-old philosophy, you have made a believer out of yourself in no time when you start to experience the power of positive thinking working inside your body to build a healthier you.

Exercise

It is an exercise that is one of the most neglected factors in healing the body. Over the years, it reduces to a fitness role, equivalent to the need to stay in shape or help achieve this goal, rather than a balanced practice in itself. Exercise releases endorphins to provide relief from pain and a sense of happiness and well-being at large.

Good diet

A balanced diet is a beautiful resource for healing your body as much as it can cause you to know it. To maintain maximum health, you need other nutrients. That's why it's essential to bear in mind other choices like vitamin supplements— although they're not nearly as successful as getting the nutrients through your diet.

Adopt Healthy Habits

Replace antibacterial soap with your regular hand soap. Often wash your hands and wash them well. Teach your family how to wash their faces, cover their mouths, and use sanitizing hand wipes or liquid cleaners in public to reduce the risk of taking home infections and diseases. Such practices can seem too simplistic but may result in prevention, which is often the best treatment, allowing the body to heal.

Protecting the Body with Hypnosis

Self-hypnosis is just another means of protecting the body from illnesses of all kinds. In many ways mastering the art of self-hypnosis can help in your struggle, whether you are trying to reject cancer that is just as hard to take over or ward off the common cold. Hypnosis can help you relax, open your mind to positive thinking, help the nutrients get where they best serve, and help boost immunity, among other great things.

Take Control of Your Healing Process

Whether you are using one or all of the above techniques, if you listen to your body and react accordingly—for the best possible health outcome—you can find real help when it comes to healing the body. Hypnosis is a powerful mode that literally can help your body stop unwanted habits and then start to heal and rejuvenate your body. It's all about the computer device situated within the brain. After about five years, smoking stops being fun, and you realize how reliant you are becoming on that smelly habit. Does anyone enjoy the desperation and mental obsession with a dried leaf filled with those little white papers that have become your best friend? It's true; it's that bad cynical friend you have to take with you everywhere you go. Those "cigs" will be with you 24 hours a day and seven days a week, and you'll want to press the panic button if, by chance, you run out. That's how it has been for me. For 30 years, I smoke tons of cigarettes a day. Before the day I was hypnotized and quit smoking forever, I knew nothing about my subconscious strength. It's why I became a Hypnotherapist, too. Stress creates the need to smoke, or does it cause anxiety? It is tough to go cold-turkey in this modern-day world where tension is a daily occurrence. Hypnotherapy is often the last option, yet smoking cessation is the most successful strategy than any prescription medication designed to quit smoking. Stress will manifest itself in all sorts of scenarios. You are ranging from being depressed to violent. Contrary to common opinion, medications just exacerbate the condition while making huge bucks for the pharmaceuticals. Seek your nearest Hypnotherapist first before you go to get medicine to be healthy again. You're going to be happier faster, and it's going to last a lot longer! Will they hypnotize you? Hey! The condition you strive to achieve is one of absolute relaxation as though you're about to fall asleep. You are still very much in charge because we enhance your drive to do what you set out to do. Hypnosis is essentially a form of deep relaxation that allows the client to take an imagined journey. The imagination is where you build a new, vibrant vision for what you want to be like in your future. When your critical mind is in a profoundly relaxed state, it calms down from that constant thinking that says: "I can't just leave," or "It's just too hard to quit." Side-stepping the critical mind lets you become motivated to accomplish what you felt was impossible before. Not only does it work well with smoking, but it also works well in sports, handling discomfort, and even taking exams. Old habits of thinking replace quickly and lovingly with fresh, wonderful optimistic thoughts that can leave such a positive force in your life. Imagine if you can avoid obsessing about a question, you can do something, be, and have anything. You broke the habit, and you can achieve anything set out to do. Your level of confidence goes sky-high! The most widespread problem is that after stopping smoking, customers assume they'll gain weight. Luckily, when the body recovers from the smoking effects, the value would inevitably result in a benefit or loss. It is a positive thing meaning that the body is in the healing process. You can also eradicate the habit with hypnosis, and stop replacing one oral obsession with another. The subconscious mind is already planting the new thought cycle, and when you listen to your private session's mp3, you can reduce the weight tension. I suggest that you choose a hypnotherapist who has your mind-rejuvenating your heart and lungs back to an age you feel tremendous strength and energy. A successful hypnotherapist can even get your liver to detoxify your body very gently so that the tar and nicotine or even heavy metals extract very quickly and easily. The body is in the healing process until they leave the workplace and remain there for a few months. Hypnotherapy will help move the body into new wellness. Your cells order to heal through the science of Epigenetics. Hypnosis is the best way to help cancer patients help the body recover faster, particularly with surgeries. Studies show hypnosis heals the body to minimize bleeding, swelling, and bruises and speed up the recovery process ten times more quickly. In addition to that, it establishes that 10 minutes of hypnosis reduce blood pressure and lower cholesterol. If you want to quit smoking, eradicate a phobia, heal cancer or pain, then just use your healthy and focused mind to seek it out without medication. It is a lot easier than you could ever imagine. You become a champion, and you'll be shocked by how strong you are.

CHAPTER 20

WHY DO WE STRUGGLE
WITH WEIGHT?

For anyone who has tried to lose weight, life seems to be an uphill battle. Seeing how difficult it is to reverse the situation and lose some weight can be downright devastating. Most of them require you to understand better why this struggle occurs and what steps you can take to win the battle. Although there may be physical factors that affect your ability to maintain excess weight Many psychological, emotional, and even spiritual reasons may affect your en- tire body's ability to help you lose weight and reach your ideal weight level. That is why this part is about focusing on those "hidden" causes, the kinds that go beyond the apparent aspects which are widely conversed in the mainstream media and by everyday folks. We will discuss how you can look inward to under-stand where and how things might need to change so that you can start to turn things around and make a positive impact on your life.

The Obvious Culprits

The obvious culprits that are holding you back are diet, a lack of exercise, and a combination of both. First off, your diet plays a crucial role in your overall health and wellbeing. When it comes to weight management, your diet has everything to do with your ability to stay in shape and ward of unwanted weight. When it comes to diet, we are not talking about keto, vegan, or Atkins; we are talking about the everyday foods you consume and their amounts. When you consume high amounts of sugar, carbs, and fats, your body transforms them into glucose, stored in the body as fat. Of course, a proportion of the glucose produced by your body uses up as energy. However, if you consume far more than you need, your body will not get rid of it; your body will hold on to it and make sure that it stores for a rainy day. If you are asking yourself why the body does that, the answer is simple. Over thousands of years of evolution, humankind has struggled to have enough to eat. It hasn't been until about the last two hundred years that most societies have abundant amounts of food. It has enabled our generations to eat three meals a day and a little more. Given that our early ancestors would go days without eating, evolution has programmed the human body to store up as much fat as possible. If the body program otherwise, it would have some sort of mechanism that would either shut off hunger or use up the fat that store up or signal the body to get somehow rid of excess fat but we're not there yet. Perhaps, the body will evolve such a response. Before that, we need to work tirelessly and understand why we gain weight in this way. Here is another crucial aspect to consider: sweet and salty foods, which we love so dearly, trigger "happy hormones" in the brain, namely dopamine. Dopamine is a hormone that is released by the body when it "feels good." It is why you somehow feel better after eating your favorite meals. It also explains the reason why we resort to food when we are not feeling well. It is called "comfort food," and it is one of the most popular coping mechanisms employed by folks worldwide. This rush of dopamine causes a person to become addicted to food. As with any addiction, there comes a time when you need to get more and more of that same substance to meet your body's requirements. It's the same as happens with a drug addict or alcoholic. They need to consume more and more of the substance they are addicted to getting the same rush. In a way, the body develops a resistance to the "happy hormones" released when eating yummy food. Therefore, you need an ever-increasing amount of these hormones for you to get your fix. The inevitable result of dieting is that lack of regular exercise can help you lose weight and maintain a healthy balance. What regular exercise does is increase your body's overall caloric requirement. As such, your metabolism needs to convert fat at higher rates to keep up with your body's energy demands. On paper, this is a relatively straightforward process. Through cellular respiration, the body converts glucose (or fat back into glucose) and combines it with oxygen to produce energy. This process makes it possible for the body to restore its caloric intake into life, thereby providing power for the body's movement. As the body's energetic requirements increase, that is, as your exercise regimen gets more and more intense, you will find that you will need increased amounts of both oxygen and glucose. It is one of the reasons why you feel hungrier when you ramp up your workouts. However, increasing your calorie intake is not just to consume more and more calories; you also need to complete the same amount of protein, carbohydrates, fats, and vitamins to make your body build necessary. These elements will strengthen muscles, promote exercise, and provide proper oxygenation for the blood.

Moreover, nutrients are required for the body to recover. One of the byproducts of exercise is called "lactic acid." Lactic acid signals the body that it is time to stop working out or risk injury if you continue. Without lactic acid, your body would have no way of knowing when your muscles have overextended their capacity. After you have completed your workout, the body needs to get rid of the lactic acid build-up. So, if you don't have enough of the right minerals in your body, for example, potassium, your muscles will ache for days until your body can finally get rid of the lactic acid buildup. This example shows how proper nutrition is needed to help the body get moving and recover once exercising. As a result, a lack of exercise reconfigures your body's metabolism to work at a slower pace. Therefore, if you eventually consume more energy than you need, your body discards on rainy days. Plain and simple.

The Sneaky Culprits

 The sneaky culprits are the ones that aren't quite so overt in causing you to gain weight or have trouble shedding pounds. These culprits hide beneath the surface but are very useful when it comes to keeping you overweight. The first culprit we are going to be looking at is called "stress."

Stress is a potent force. From an evolutionary perspective, it exists as a means of fueling the flight-or-fight response. Focus is the human response to danger. When a person senses danger, the body begins to secrete a hormone called "cortisol." When cortisol begins running through the body, it signals the entire system to prep for a potential showdown. Depending on the situation, it's best to tail it and fight for another day. Regardless of the outcome, the main point is to ensure survival. This evolutionary trait is what has helped preserve the human species throughout thousands of years. In modern life, though, stress plays a very different role. In our modern way of life, stress isn't so much a response to life and death situations (though it can certainly be); instead, it responds to problems deemed "conflictive" by the mind. It could be a confrontation with a co-worker, bumper to bumper traffic, or any other type of situation in which a person feels vulnerable in some way. Throughout our lives, we subject to countless interactions in which we must deal with stress. In general terms, the feelings of alertness subside when the perceived threat is gone. One such change is overexposure to cortisol. When there is too much cortisol in the body, the body's overall response is to accumulate calories, increase other hormones (such as adrenaline), and enhance the immune system's function.   This response by the body is akin to the panic response that the body would assume when faced with prolonged periods of hunger or fasting. As a result, the body needs to go into survival mode. Please bear in mind that the body has no clue if it is being chased by a bear, dealing with a natural disaster, or just having a bad day at the office. Regardless of the circumstances, the body faces the need to en- sure its survival. So, anything that it eats goes straight to fat stores.   Moreover, a person's stressful situation makes them search for comfort and solace. There are various means of achieving this. Food is one of them. So is alcohol consumption. These two types of amenities lead to high consumption of calories. Your body has been under tremendous pressure It what makes you gain weight when you are stressed out Now, suppose you go on a low-carb crash diet. Your body has been under tremendous pressure. On top of that, you choose to take away its usual caloric in- take. What do you think will be the body's response? A further deepening of its panic mode. It is the main reason why crash diets only partially work.   Another of the sneaky culprits is sleep deprivation. In short, sleep deprivation is sleeping less than the recommended 8 hours that all adults should sleep. In the children's cases, the recommended amount of sleep can be anywhere from 8 to 12 hours, depending on their age.   Granted, some adults can function perfectly well with less than 8 hours' sleep. Some folks can work perfectly well with 6 hours' sleep while shattered folks don't get eight or even more hours' sleep. It is different for everyone, as each individual is different in this regard. That says sleep deprivation can trigger massive amounts of cortisol. It, fueled by ongoing exposure to stress, leads the body to further deepening its panic mode.

CHAPTER 21

MAINTENANCE AND DAILY EXERCISES

Keep a Journal

Traveling is a healthy habit for many people, regardless of their goals, but it is essential for those who want to lose weight. By writing down your different portion measurements and exercise habits, you can better ensure that you'll have a basis for evaluation. A food diary puts into the record circumstances that lead to eating, what eats, and what amounts. Also include the feelings before, during, and after eating. This way, one can keep track of eating habits and emotions. It helps in determining the patterns of behaviors surrounding food. It will be the basis for making adjustments and designing treatments.

Stress management

Stress is one trigger that cannot remove from one's life. Stress will happen, in varying degrees, at different times of the day, in different situations. Learning to deal, tolerate, and manage stress is most important to keep binge eating under control.

Regular eating schedule

Commit and stick to the meal schedules. Regardless of what happens in the day (or night), make sure to keep to the eating schedule. Otherwise, one might soon go back to unhealthy eating habits and attitudes. For example, skipping breakfast would mean low energy during the more significant part of the morning.

Stay away from temptation

Get rid of the foods and stay away from situations that trigger binge eating. Re- move all junk foods, unhealthy snacks, and desserts from the home, office, car, etc. Binge eaters are good at hiding food. Practically, every nook and cranny uses to hide food, including closets, drawers, and even the floorboards. Get rid of all this stash. Remove all favorite binge foods.

Live an active lifestyle and get some regular exercise

Exercise is a great way to start feeling good. It is known to stimulate the release of feel-good hormones. It brings hormonal balance and metabolism back to nor- mal levels and rates. It lifts depression and reduces the amount of stress in the body. The mood improves and curbs the urge for emotional eating. Health improves, and soon, one can see improvements in physical appearance. These changes help me feel better about the self and are more motivated to live a healthy life.

Avoid boredom

Most people snack on unhealthy foods when they feel bored. They munch on chips and other junk foods when they have nothing to do. Engage in distracting but healthy, positive activities. The change in scenery can be a distraction in itself. Or try a new hobby such as gardening, painting, or other crafts. These activities help in fighting boredom while remaining productive. Seeing the results of these activities also adds to feeling better about the self. The sense of accomplishment from these activities can boost self-esteem.

Get good quality sleep

Sleep should be restful and at regular hours. I feel tired due to a lack of enough drive to keep eating despite not feeling hungry or full. The body attempts to keep a steady supply of energy to sustain activities. If this is the case, take a power nap. Close your eyes and rest for 15 minutes at lunchtime or during the afternoon break to replenish energy, not to eat. If power naps are not possible, go to bed earlier to catch up on much-needed sleep.

Learn to listen and follow what the body is saying

Be more attuned to body signals. When it comes to hunger, learn to differentiate physical needs from emotional hunger. Physical hunger is hunger because the body has not had anything to eat for quite some time.

Get adequate social support

Whether from family, relatives, friends, coworkers, community members, or binge eaters' support groups, get others involved in the treatments.

Encourage to seek help

Waiting too long before seeing help may cause more problems. Diseases are likely to develop due to bingeing patterns, such as heart problems and obesity. En- courage the loved one to seek professional. Better yet, offer to accompany them to a health professional.

Eat right

The effectiveness of your diet depends on the quality of the food you eat. Be sure to eat foods that help you lose fat and give you essential nutrients to reach your weight loss goal.

Drink right

Water is essential in promoting good health. People who consume water tend to be healthier and happier than people who don't drink water. Also, drinking water will help to prevent you from certain diseases. You can also consume water by eating food that has a lot of water in them like watermelon. The highest percentage of food is composed of water, so you are also consuming water as you consume food. If you're not used to drinking water in the glass cup, then you can start with one or two glasses a day and increase it every day. If you don't love drinking water, then look for things that will put in the situation to drink water. For instance, you might decide to gift yourself something after consuming a certain amount of water for the day. Drinking water isn't a big deal, and you can train yourself to drink water daily. Meditation will help you maintain the focus you need to drink the water level you need each day. It will help you to create a plan for drinking water and to stick to that plan. Water has zero calories. If you drink it cold, you will burn more calories because your body heats it to internal temperature. Best of all, it's available almost everywhere. If plain water bores you, take it sparkled, or with a slice of lemon, cucumber, or apple for a more refreshing drink.

Tweak Your Lifestyle

Every little thing counts. It is an important thing to note if you want to lose weight and slim down. Making a few changes in your regular daily activities can help you burn more calories.

Rest

Your mind and body need rest. Excessive work on your body leads to muscle atrophy and unnecessary stress on your system. You need adequate sleep for mus- cle recovery and for your subconscious mind to process and work on things.

CHAPTER 22

WHAT ARE AFFIRMATIONS?

AFFIRMATIONS ARE POSITIVE statements used to challenge and overcome nega- tive thoughts. They can increase motivation and help you accomplish goals. Re- peating and believing them can help you begin to make positive changes to your life.

Instructions

PLEASE FOLLOW THESE guidelines carefully in order to ensure your comfort and safety.

1. It's best to listen to the audiobook in a private, comfortable environment where you won't be disturbed for at least fifteen to thirty minutes. There's no wrong time, but never listen when your attention is required elsewhere. For your safety, don't listen while driving, cycling, operating machinery, or handling sharp objects.

2. For maximum positive benefits, listen to the audiobook every day at first.

3. You can slowly reduce this to every other day. The time frame is different for everyone, so it's vital to listen frequently, to begin with, and find what works for you as time goes on.

4. It's suggested that you listen to the audiobook with

headphones on to eliminate any distractions and increase your focus on the words. For a higher chance of success, keep an open mind. Concentrate on positive thoughts and feelings. All you need to do is let go, relax, and enjoy.

5. Make sure you are comfortable. Lie down on a soft surface, such as a bed, or sit in a comfy seat. You can even invest in a meditation chair or pillow, along with an eye mask if you are listening while lying down.

The Difference Between Guided Meditation and Guided Hypnosis

GUIDED MEDITATION AND hypnosis are very similar. Both can be used for sonal growth. However, there are a few differences. Mediation is a form of training your mind and is commonly labeled as the absence of thought. It's used to obtain a higher sense of relaxation. It can awaken a sense of inner calm by quieting your mind and helping you focus. Hypnosis, on the other hand, is a way of selective thinking to accomplish specific results. It puts you in a state of altered consciousness, making you more open to suggestions. Contrary to popular belief, hypnosis is not the lack of control but is an enhanced sense of control and awareness. As such, both are completely safe and have been proven to yield many benefits.

CHAPTER 23

SHORT GUIDED MEDITATION

Short Guided Meditation 1 (15 Mins)
Relaxation

THIS SESSION IS A SHORTER one meant to be listened to on weekdays when you have less time to dedicate to these sessions. It will be around fifteen minutes long. This may be difficult to manage at first but don't worry. You can take it slowly, one breath at a time. If you only manage a few minutes this time, you can manage a few more tomorrow and a few more the day after that. This session is all about relaxation. Start by making sure you are comfortable.

Find a quiet place to lie down or sit. You will want your back to be straight but relax your posture and shoulders. Close your eyes. Take a deep breath through your nose, loosening all your muscles and joints. Let the breath out through your mouth, letting go of it as though you were blowing your stress away. I want you to think about the feelings going through your body. Make sure that your back, your shoulders, and your neck are comfortable. Roll your ankles and your wrists before relaxing them as well. Wiggle your fingertips and your toes, loosening them. If you are sitting, make sure your feet are flat on the ground, feeling the energy of the earth beneath you. Once you are relaxed and comfortable, you are going to concentrate on breathing again. Rest one hand comfortably on your stomach, just below your rib cage, and one on your upper chest. Just like before, I want you to breathe in slowly and deeply through your nose so that your stomach moves out against your hand. Afterward, breathe out through your mouth. The hand on your chest should move as little as possible. Keep doing this technique. Breathe in deeply. Breathe out, allowing all the air and stress to leave you. This session is all about relaxation. You are going to try and release all of that tension that you may not even know your muscles have been holding onto. This be- gins with your body, and we will move on to your mind. While you listen to my voice, keep breathing in and out. Concentrate on doing this.

Inhale deeply through your nose, then exhale through your mouth. You should already be beginning to feel more relaxed. If you are, you are going to move on to relaxing your body. You will start from your head and move down the rest of your body until we eventually reach your toes. Start by tensing the muscles in your face and scalp. Inhale and hold this for the count of five. I want you to pull your face into a tight frown, shutting your eyes as tightly as you can and gritting your teeth. If you can move your ears up and down to tighten your scalp, you should do so.

Once you have reached five, let go of all the tension. You are going to exhale and let your face go completely slack. Take your time with this before we move onto the next step. Feel the strain trickling from your facial muscles. Indulge in that feeling. If you need to, you can repeat until your face feels completely relaxed. Now, I want you to move on to your neck. Tense your neck and shoulders.

Once again, inhale and count to five. Once you reach your count, exhale and relax your neck and shoulders. Roll them to loosen the joints just like you did at the start of the session. Many people carry the majority of their tension in their neck and shoulders, so if you feel like you need to, you can repeat this step too. Take your time and let your- self go completely. You want to make sure that all your muscles are relaxed and loose. Remain calm and breathe as you go. You are going to work your way down from your neck to all the major muscle groups.

Tighten your arms and pull your forearms up to your bicep before stretching them back out again. Clench your hands into fists and then loosen them again, wiggling your fingers. Roll your wrists. Roll your hips. Pull your knees up but don't push it past the point of comfort. Stretch them out again. Lastly, clench your toes just like you did with your fingers and loosen them again. Roll your ankles. Remember, you can repeat each muscle group until it feels completely relaxed.

Finally, I want you to breathe again. Concentrate on breathing only now. Inhale deeply through your nose, then exhale through your mouth.

By now, you should feel more relaxed and able to return to your day.

Short Guided Meditation 2 (15 Mins)
Stop Overthinking, Anxiety, and Stress

THIS SESSION IS A SHORTER one meant to be listened to on weekdays when you have less time to dedicate to these sessions. It will be around fifteen minutes long. This is the second session. If you find it difficult, you still have the option of doing it for a few minutes and gradually increasing the time as you go on. You can take it slowly, one breath at a time. This session is about stopping overthinking, anxiety, and stress. Start by making sure you are comfortable.

Find a quiet place to lie down or sit. You will want your back to be straight but relax your posture and shoulders. Close your eyes. Take a deep breath through your nose, loosening all your muscles and joints. Let the breath out through your mouth, letting go of it as though you were blowing your stress away. Think about the feelings of your body. Allow yourself to feel every inch. Make sure that your back, your shoulders, and your neck are comfortable. You can roll your neck and shoulders for this part. Roll your ankles and your wrists before relaxing them. Wiggle your fingertips and your toes, loosening them as well. If you are sit- ting, make sure your feet are flat on the ground, feeling the energy of the earth beneath you. Allow this energy to course through your body and calm you. Continue with the breathing technique. Breathe in deeply.

Breathe out, allowing all the air and stress to leave you. Rest a hand on your belly and feel it push out against your hand as you breathe in through your nose. Breathe out through your mouth again, allowing your stomach to fall flat. You are going to try to clear your mind this time. The practice here is not to have no thoughts at all. That would be incredibly difficult. Instead of trying to have no thoughts, I want you to let them pass through your mind, but try not to hold onto any of them. Right now, I want you to imagine that your mind is a clear blue sky and thoughts are nothing more than wispy clouds passing through.

Have you ever watched the clouds? If you have, you might have tried to recognize shapes out of them. Perhaps some clouds simply stuck out to you more than others. One thing we know about clouds is that they are always on the move. They don't stay in one place. They float along with the breeze, moving along the blue sky until eventually, you can no longer watch them. You have to move on to the next cloud or turn away from them altogether. This is how I want you to picture your thoughts. Your mind is going to be clear as a blue sky. If any thoughts drift show up, let them. Just like a cloud, they will only drift through your mind. They are white and fluffy and light. Let them go by without concentrating or paying too much attention to them, and when they start to disappear, don't hold onto them.

All the while, remember to breathe gently in and out. Letting your breathing be- come the first priority can help distract you from wandering thoughts. Concentrate on taking deep breaths in and out. Next, I want you to picture any stress and anxiety you might have. Imagine that your worries, whatever they may be, are a tangible thing. Perhaps there's something at work or at home stressing you out and making you anxious. This time, instead of clouds, I want you to picture those things taking form in the shape of playdough. You can choose the color of the dough. Make the stresses at home green, the stresses at work red, and so on. You can choose whatever colors you feel most comfortable with. Picture the dough in your hands, malleable and breakable. You can squash it between your fingertips and feel that it's wet and soft. It's almost like a stress ball as you gently close your hands around it and release it. Imagine that you can break small pieces off and squish them between your fingers until the playdough gets smaller and smaller. Soon it becomes a manageable size and practically disappears. Break it up into smaller pieces until eventually there is nothing left. Continue to breathe in and out while you do this. Let go of all the negative thoughts and feelings. Let them seep from your pores for a healthier and more positive mind.

Slowly, I want you to open your eyes and return to your day.

Short Guided Meditation 3 (15 Mins)
Relaxation, Stop Thinking, Deep Sleep

THIS SESSION IS A SHORTER one meant to be listened to on weekdays when you have less time to dedicate to these sessions. It will be around fifteen minutes long. This is the third session. Hopefully, you are finding it easier to manage the amount of time dedicated to meditation around now. Each minute should be taken slowly. This session is about relaxation, stop thinking, deep sleep. Just like before, you are going to start out by making sure that you are comfortable in a quiet place. You will want to make sure that the lights are either off or dimmed this time. There should be no harsh lighting to make it easier for you to drift off. I want you to lie down on a soft, comfortable surface, whether that is a bed or a sofa or a meditation mat. Keep your back straight but relax your shoulders and posture. Loosen all your muscles and joints, relaxing your body completely, before you start breathing. Take a deep breath in through your nose and let it out through your mouth, letting go of anything you were doing before.

Put yourself in the cur- rent moment, forgetting about all the worries of yesterday, today, and tomorrow. None of those matters right now. All you need to do is relax and continue to breathe in and out. Slow and steady. In and out. Deep breaths in through your nose and gentle breaths out through your mouth. There may be thoughts circling around inside your mind. I want you to focus on them but don't hold onto them. Your thoughts are going to be like small birds gliding back and forth through your mind. They will have feathers, soft and smooth, but they don't have voices. They are silent and calm as they slowly float around. Imagine that the birds have a color, something light and relaxing. You can watch as the small birds flutter to and fro inside your mind but don't try to catch them. Let them be free. Allow them to fly away from you. Let them shrink into the distance as they slowly drift away from you, the gentle wind of their wings taking any stress with them as they go. They are leaving behind a calm, serene environment for you to enjoy.

Breathe in through your nose and out through your mouth. Take deep and calming breaths and let go of them easily. Your body is loose and relaxed. You can feel every inch of it beginning to get heavy where it touches the soft surface beneath you. At this moment, you are feeling calm and comfortable with each breath you take. As you inhale, you invite peace and harmony into your life. Nothing matters but this moment where you breathe in and out. As you exhale, you release the day and all the stresses that came with it. Your mind is becoming more relaxed too. Picture the ocean, deep blue-green color with a tinge of white foam on its surface. It's early morning, and the sun glistens off of the water like tiny diamonds as it flows with its own current. The waves are crashing gently on the shore before being taken back by the sea. Allow yourself to be taken by your mind like a gentle guide, the same way the ocean pulls on the waves as they crash forward onto the beach. It lulls you, the same way the sea ebbs and flows onto the sand with a gentle crash of the waves. Imagine that soft whooshing sound and the refreshing feeling that comes with sea air on your skin. Backward and forward the waves go, slowly and gently. If any thoughts return, remember the birds from before. They will flutter and glide high above you, over the ocean in a clear blue sky. Pay attention to the gentle lull of the ocean. Worry not over the birds in the sky. They have no voice. Let them quietly drift across the sky and away from you. As the thoughts drift away, becoming smaller and smaller until they finally disappear into the distance, your mind begins to feel like a clear and serene environment. You breathe in and out in a gentle rhythm with the waves of the ocean. In and out, the same way the waves crash back and forth. Your body feels heavy and relaxed. You can let go of it and let it drift.

If you are still awake, turn the listening device off. You are so sleepy by this point that you will fall asleep as soon as you close your eyes again. You will wake up feeling fresh and rejuvenated after a good night's rest.

Short Guided Meditation 4 (15 Mins)
Relaxation

THIS IS A FIFTEEN-MINUTE session to help put you in a state of relaxation. You are going to start this session by making sure that you are nice and comfortable. Find a quiet place to sit where you won't be disturbed for at least fifteen minutes. Bring yourself to the here and now. Nothing else matters but this present moment. Close your eyes and breathe. That's all you have to do right now. You just need to breathe. I want you to rest a hand on your belly and take a deep breath in. Don't hold it. Keep it as natural as possible. Right now, your breath is like the branches and leaves of a tree blowing in a gentle breeze. You are the tree. You go with nature, not against it.

Simply feel your belly slowly expanding beneath your hand. When you breathe out, feel the way it goes flat. That's the feeling of tension leaving your body. With each breath you take, you are inviting a gentle feeling of relaxation into yourself, and each time you breathe out, you are releasing all the negativity from your mind and body. Take deep breaths in through your nose and release them out through your mouth. Calm yourself with each slow breath, in and out, again and again. You are inviting peace and calmness to your body and mind. Most of us hold a lot of tension in our jaw without even knowing it. I want you to make sure that this isn't the case for you. Slowly, I want you to open your mouth as wide as you can without hurting yourself.

Hold your mouth open for at least ten seconds, breathing naturally through your nose, before closing it again. I want you to repeat this motion three times. Stretch your jaw out. When you close your mouth for the third time, you should notice that your face feels more relaxed. Follow this motion by rolling your neck in one direction and then doing the same in the opposite direction. Do it slowly, pulling your head back- ward and forward, from side to side. Your eyes should still be closed. Remember to keep breathing in and out, deeply. Feel the way your belly pushes against your palm while you roll your head. Your muscles should be feeling much looser and more relaxed. Let go and place yourself at this moment. You are taking time off for yourself right now. The only thing you need to think about is the gentle, soothing breaths in and out and the softness of the comfortable thing your body is on. Rest your head backward. Let it relax against the gentle pillow behind it. Imagine that the pillow is a sponge, and it's soaking up all the worries of the day. Allow your head to sink into the soft cushioning and release all of it. It's being drawn away from you by the relaxing and comfortable space that you have put yourself into. Release all the negative energy of the day and only keep the positive vibes. Feel the positivity running through your body, each nerve tingling with the soothing sensation of goodness.

You are feeling better about the fact that you have set this time aside to center and balance yourself. Your calm breaths in and out are helping refresh your body, in and out. You are making an effort to better yourself by being here and soothing your mind and body.

Move your hands and gently rest them at your sides. Your arms should be loose and relaxed. No part of your body should be tense right now. Slacken your body. All you have to do right now is simply be. Stretch your fingers and your toes out with each breath in, loosening the tension that you are holding onto, and gently curl them in with each breath out. Stretch out. Curl in. Gently. Do this with each breath you take. Your whole body should be feeling light and rejuvenated. Stop stretching your fingers and toes. You can let them go slack, along with the rest of your body. All I want you to do is let the cushioning beneath your body draw out all the worries and tired feelings of the day. Breathe in and out. Let the relaxation take you away from here. Follow the breeze where it takes you, lulling your body.

When you open your eyes, you should be ready to face your day with a renewed sense of energy.

Short Guided Meditation 5 (15 Mins)
Stop Overthinking, Anxiety, and Stress

THIS IS A FIFTEEN-MINUTE session to help you overcome overthinking, stress, and anxiety. The best way to stop you from overthinking is to practice mindfulness. This is not a small thing that you can do once or twice. Mindfulness is something that is going to take time and dedication for it to work effectively. Don't worry though. You are practicing mindfulness just by making an effort to listen to my voice on a regular basis. Following my guidance and taking the things you hear into account are ways of moving forward to a better you and a more peaceful future. To stop your- self from overthinking, you need to become more aware of the present time. That's what we are going to do in this session. We are going to practice awareness. Start by sitting or lying down. Make yourself comfortable but keep your back straight. Your posture should be relaxed, but you should be alert. Make sure that you aren't straining in any way. Your clothes, muscles, and joints should not be tense. Close your eyes and think about your body. Notice the way that it feels, the still- ness of it, and the relaxed sensation of your chest and shoulders. Loosen your body. Let go of the tension. Let your shoulders go slack, rest your head back, and unclench your jaw. You are going to start breathing now. Breathe in deeply through your nose, letting your diaphragm expand with the breath, and then slowly release. Repeat this technique, allowing the air to gently flow through your body and a sense of calm wash over you from head to toe. I want you to release the stress and anxiety that have been plaguing you. Find a comfortable rhythm to breathe in and out. Understand that your thoughts will wander. This is natural. While not all your thoughts and feelings will be good, it's important to let them pass by. Watch them from a distance, as an outsider looking in. Picture yourself on a bus. It's a comfortable, quiet bus, and you are the only passenger on your way to a tranquil environment.

The bus is driving through the countryside. Greenery surrounds you from all sides, and it is a beautiful clear day. There are no clouds in the sky, and the sun shines down on you, warming your face with its gentle rays and making you feel invigorated. When thoughts come into your mind, imagine that you are passing flowers in a field. The thoughts are nothing but flowers in a meadow. You can't smell their scent because the windows are closed, but you can see their colors. Give each feeling a color and notice the way the field is alive with it. Don't try to look back as you glance out of the window. Allow the bus to continue driving, passing the colorful flowers and leaving them behind. This is what you are going to do with your thoughts. They are seeds, planting flowers that grow in the greenery of your mind, but you don't need to pay them much heed right now. All you need to do is concentrate on breathing in and out, going with the flow. Enjoy the drive and relax as you pass through the beautiful countryside on either side of you. Eventually, you will leave the flowers, your thoughts, behind. Keep breathing in and out. You can notice and acknowledge the flowers but don't follow them. Don't let your mind pursue them. You don't need to look back at them. Simply let them pass by you. You are on your bus, driving away from the flowers as they disappear into the distance behind you. Let go of them as you breathe. You are moving forward with the bus as you breathe, inhaling deeply through your nose and exhaling gently through your mouth. The flowers are going to blow and flow in the breeze, and that's okay. They will do that. Flowers grow in meadows, and there's nothing you can do about it. But you can choose to leave them there. You don't need to stare, you don't need to pick them, and you don't need to smell their scent. Instead, continue to move through them, allowing you to simply pass through their path.

When you are ready, the bus will start to slow down, and you will be able to step off of it. Slowly, open your eyes and stand up. You can stretch your limbs out, feeling refreshed and energized to return to your day.

Short Guided Meditation 6 (15 Mins)
Relaxation, Stop Thinking, Deep Sleep

THIS IS A FIFTEEN-MINUTE session to relax you, help you stop thinking, and allow you to drift off into a deep sleep. All the lights should be turned off and dimmed to create a more tranquil environment. You should be lying down. You can lie down on a bed, a sofa, or a meditation mat. The most important part is to make sure that you are comfortable and relaxed, ready to drift off into a deep sleep, where no one will disturb you. Your body should be slack and loose. All of your muscles and joints should be drooping as you let go of yourself. You are letting yourself relax completely. As always, you are going to start breathing. Breathe in deeply through your nose and breathe out gently through your mouth. As you breathe, release all the tension of the day. Let the stress and excitement ooze from your pores and bones, draining all the negative energy from your mind and body. You have only good feelings at this moment, the comforting feel of a soft cushion beneath your body as it draws the energy from you.

Concentrate on and give yourself to the current moment. Your day is coming to an end, and it's time to settle into a deep and restful night. You are going to let go of every bad thing, feeling, and thought that you have from today. None of that matters. All that matters right now is this second where you rest and the feelings that are going through your body right now. While you breathe in, your belly pushes outward, and each time you breathe out, you clear your thoughts. Let your chest rise and gently fall with each slow and steady breath. These breaths are clearing your body and mind of all unhealthy feelings and thoughts, replacing them with positivity. If there are any thoughts in your mind right now, don't try to fight their presence. They are supposed to be there. They belong in your mind. Instead of concentrating on them, let them be. Right now, your thoughts are going to be like those floating transparent bubbles. You know those little bubbles in a bottle that kids have? They blow bubbles through a wand, and then rainbow-colored bubbles float through the air. And they can be popped, or they float higher and higher into the air until they finally vanish beyond our sight. That is what is going to happen with your thoughts. Each time a stray thought drifts through the clarity of your mind, it's going to be nothing more than a bubble blown through. They're empty and glow slightly with their rainbow colors where the light touches them.

Instead of reaching out to try and catch or pop the bubbles, you're going to simply let them float away from you. Watch as they go higher and higher until eventually they're gone. Breathe in and out while you watch. If you inhale deeply enough, you might find that the bubbles move toward you almost like you're sucking them in. If you ex- hale, you blow them away from you. This is going to work to clear your mind even more. It will be a calming and soothing environment for you to rest in. Give your mind a background color. This color is going to be the color of your relaxation. You can choose anything you feel comfortable with. The color of lavenders, a light purple, or the color of freshly mown grass, bright green, are both good colors to think about. The longer you rest in this serene color, the easier you feel. Your breaths are light and relaxed. Your body is letting go of everything and becoming heavier and heavier against the soft surface beneath your body. Your eyelids are heavy, and you can't bring yourself to open them. Behind your eyelids, you can see the color you were thinking of. Any thoughts are still bubbles, empty and light as they drift across the background. You can feel yourself drifting off with the thoughts, falling into a deep sleep. The feeling of your own gentle breathing lulls you into a state of serene clarity. In and out, slow and steady, you breathe deeply and gently. It's like a soothing lullaby, gently guiding you into the embrace of a warm and kind night of sleep.

Your arms, legs, hands, feet, and neck all feel heavy as you give yourself over to your dreams. If you are still awake, you can turn the device off. When you close your eyes again, you'll find that you easily drift into a deep sleep.

CHAPTER 24

LONG GUIDED MEDITATION

Long Guided Meditation 1 (30 Mins)

Relaxation

THIS SESSION IS A LONGER one meant to be listened to when you have more time to dedicate to your meditation sessions. You can listen to this session over the weekend or while you are on holiday. It will be around thirty minutes long. By now, I am sure you have grown accustomed to your shorter sessions.

They have either already gotten or are beginning to get easier to sit through. You've found that you can go for longer periods of time. These longer sessions may take a little get- ting used to once again. As before, you are welcome to take these sessions slowly, one breath at a time. If you only manage half the session or a little more than half the session, that's okay. You can always take on a little more next time. And you can try a little more the time after that. This session is all about relaxation. Listen to my voice and allow your mind to lull into a peaceful state. Let yourself follow a state of pure serenity, letting go of every- thing but the calming sensations dancing through your body. You are going to start out by making sure that you are comfortable. You can lie down or sit but make sure that you are in a comfortable and quiet environment where you will not be disturbed for at least thirty minutes. Keep your back straight but loosen your shoulders and neck, relaxing your posture, and letting your limbs go slack.

Once you are comfortable in a peaceful environment, close your eyes. You're going to start your breathing technique. Breathe in deeply through your nose and then breathe out gently. Let go of all the tension in your body. You are going to let yourself float into a deep relaxation. You're going to use the progressive muscle relaxation that you went through in the first short relaxation session. This is going to help your body feel looser and more relaxed than before. Begin with your face, by tightening the muscles in your face and pulling it into a grimace. Purse your lips and scrunch your eyes as tightly as you can. Clench your jaw. Hold this as you breathe in deeply for the count of five before you let go of the expression and let your face go slack.

Exhale and release all of the tension. Indulge in the feeling of all your muscles releasing the strain. If you feel like this is relaxing or you want to do it again, you are more than welcome to do so. Keep repeating until your face feels completely relaxed. Once you are ready to move on from your face, you can move down to other muscles on your face. Breathe in deeply through your nose and exhale gently through your mouth. Let your body rise and fall with the gentle motion of your breaths. You're releasing all the tension that your body holds as you breathe. Tighten and release other muscles in your body until they feel relaxed. Hold your shoulders tightly for five seconds while you inhale before releasing them, letting go of the tension as you exhale. Move on to your arms and your wrists. Work your way down your body. All the while, breathe in and out deeply. You can do this with the muscles in your thighs and your calves. Breathe in deeply.

Hold the muscle tightly for the count of five.

Five.

Four.

Three.

Two.

One.

Breathe out gently, releasing your muscles. They should be feeling much looser than before. Move onto your ankles. Roll them around in one direction before rolling them in the opposite direction. Curl your toes and stretch them out. You can do this at the same time as your fingers. Take a deep and steadying breath in. Five. Curl your fingers and toes together. Four. Clench them tightly. Three. Two. Hold this and take notice of the way that your chest and belly swell with the breath. One. Stretch your fingers and toes out as you exhale, letting go of the breath you held. Give in to the way your chest feels lighter than before. Your limbs are feeling much more relaxed. You're in a calm environment. Your whole body is growing more and more comfortable with the breath that you take. Clear your mind of all thoughts. This isn't a quick and easy feat. Take your time and allow your thoughts to leave you. They're going to drift away, and instead of trying to hold onto them, you're going to let them go where they're going. Don't follow or try to chase them. Simply allow them to carry on without you. Imagine that you are in a desert. You are in no danger here. You are in a cool, comfortable environment, but you can see the desert all around you. There are dunes in every direction, and as you watch, a gentle breeze blows across the hills and mountains of sand. The small grains blow through the air. Watch as they float through the sky, creating pathways on the surface of the sand. Enjoy the sight of the patterns that nature creates all on its own. Breathe in, ing as the earth remains unchanged. Breathe out, watching as the wind once again blows through the air. You are a force of nature in this place. You are calm and serene. The environment shifts with you. Your breaths add to the flow of this beautiful place as the sun shines down on you. You bask in its warmth, knowing that it cannot harm you because you are one with the earth. You move with it, and it moves with you. The gentle rhythm of your breathing matches the gentle breeze blowing the sand. Imagine the feeling of the warm sand beneath your bare feet. If you curl your toes, you can feel the grains between them. When you release your toes, the sand washes over your feet. It is smooth and soft, and your feet sink easily into its depth with each step you take. You go with it, giving in to the heaviness of your legs as your feet sink into the sand underfoot. Breathe in deeply through your nose as you take one step forward. Exhale out of your mouth as your foot sinks into the sand. Breathe in as you take another step. Exhale as your foot sinks.

You can feel the breeze now because you are moving with it. It's gentle, and the sand doesn't hurt your skin. Instead, it caresses every inch of you. You give in to the sensation of the warm grains against you. They blow away all the stress and tension of the day, removing the layer of negativity that sits atop your skin. Keep going with this motion. One of the ways that you can relax is by listening to soothing music or white noise. You can even listen to this while you are meditating. The sounds will block out all the noise of the world and take you even further into a state of relaxation. Imagine that you sit down in the sand just the slightest amount, like a deep cushion beneath you. Your feet are buried in the grains, feeling heavy because they're covered by the sand. Move your hands to your sides, and as you stretch your fingers outward, you feel the grains of sand. They're warm and soft. Curl your fingers inward, feeling the sand between them. Breathe in deeply as you stretch your fingers out, and breathe out gently as you curl them in.

As you listen to this, you're starting to feel refreshed. Your thoughts float by you like grains of sand, grazing your skin but leaving you behind as they move on. You keep your eyes closed and let them. You accept that these grains exist in the desert and don't try to stop them. You are simply at peace, happy to be where you are and comfortable in the sand. The longer you sit here, the more you sink into the earth. You let it take you, feeling yourself become one with it. This moment feels more natural than anything, and you simply breathe and allow yourself to feel like you are a part of it. Slowly, you're going to stand up from the stand. Feel the day begin to return to your body. You can stretch your limbs out. Wiggle your fingertips and our toes, nerves tingling as they come back to life. You're returning to yourself, and you can slowly open your eyes up and take note of your current surroundings. Take a deep breath in and release it. Repeat this motion. Breathe in deeply, feeling your stomach push outward as your body soaks up the oxygen. Breathe out, letting go of it and the mediation session. You are feeling refreshed.

You can stand up and stretch your body out before returning to your day once more. Your center realigned after taking the time to meditate.

Long Guided Meditation 2 (30 Mins)
Stop Overthinking, Anxiety, and Stress

THIS IS A LONGER SESSION meant to be listened to when you have more time on your hands to dedicate to your meditation sessions. You can listen to this one over the weekend or while you are on holiday, even if you go away. It will be around half an hour long.

By now, I am sure you have grown familiar with the shorter sessions. They have either already gotten or are beginning to get easier to sit through. You may have found that you can listen for longer periods of time. These longer sessions may take a little getting used to once again. As before, you can take these sessions slowly, one breath and one moment at a time. If you only manage half the session or a little more than half the session, that's okay. You can always take on a little more next time. And you can try a little more the time after that. This session is going to help you stop overthinking and reduce your stress and anxiety. I am going to give you some tips to do this. Listen to the sound of my voice as I guide you through this session, and we take you to a place where all that stress and anxiety can no longer affect you negatively. Find a comfortable place where you can listen to the session while you are sitting or lying down. You are going to start out by making sure that you are comfortable. You should be in a peaceful, quiet atmosphere where you will not be disturbed for at least half an hour. Keep your back straight relax your posture, resting your shoulders and neck against the cushioning behind you. Once you

GastricBand Hypnosis

are comfortable in this peaceful environment, let your eyes fall shut. Slowly, you're going to start to breathe deeply in and out. Breathe in deeply through your nose and then breathe out gently. Let go of all the tension in your body. Know that anxiety and stress exist. However, you have the choice of letting that take control of you. You are the key to releasing all of that negative energy. All it takes is time and commitment. Yet again, you're going to practice mindfulness. You're going to concentrate on being right here in the present moment. Nothing else matters but this very session. Don't worry over the future and let go of the past. This is easier said than done, but if you practice paying attention to the present, it will get much easier to do. Breathe in deeply. Breathe out gently. Release all the tension from your body. I want you to imagine that you're in a park, either sitting on a bench or lying on the grass. You are surrounded by green grass and trees. The breeze whistles through them, making the leaves and branches blow gently. The grass is spongy beneath you, soft and cool against your skin. It yields to you, making you feel like you are a part of it. Breathe in, inhaling the calm scent of the nature that surrounds you. Breathe out again. Breathe in, inviting peace and harmony to this space. Breathe out again. You may find that your thoughts are wandering. This is okay. I want you to picture that the park you're in has dandelions. You reach out, and your fingers gently brush the furry stems of the plants. Feel the softness of them. Let your whole body luxuriate in the softness of nature. Let that comfort overwhelm every inch of your body. These dandelions are your thoughts. They belong in the park that is your mind. There is nothing wrong with them, but sometimes, you may feel like the park is better off without them. I want you to reach out and pluck one of them from the ground. Imagine that this is exactly what you would do when you notice a thought that you don't really like. You can pluck it right out of your mind.

Concentrate on your breathing. If you're holding onto one of those thoughts, I want you to pay as little attention to it as possible. Breathe in deeply, clearing your mind instead. When you exhale, I want you to imagine blowing the dandelion seeds off of the head of that little plant. Watch as they blow away from you, drifting off into the sky. This is what will happen with your thoughts. You'll pick them up and then let go of them. They'll simply break apart, becoming smaller and smaller, and then eventually, they'll disappear altogether. If we make an effort to break our thoughts up into more manageable chunks, they don't seem so bad anymore. In fact, they seem a lot easier to handle. Instead of thinking about this huge dandelion you're holding onto, take note of the little seeds that there are. You plant those seeds. You have full control over where they go. Right now, you're going to let go of them. Breathe in deeply. Breathe out. Can you feel the way your chest swells with the breath? You can feel the sensation spreading throughout the fibers of your muscles. Breathe in again. Your belly expands with the breath. When you exhale, your body feels rejuvenated with the oxygen. Each time a stray thought drifts through your mind, picture that dandelion. Picture that your mind is a park, and you have the ability to pluck flowers right from the ground if you want to. Each time you exhale, you blow those seeds through the air, releasing them from your park. Here, you are in total control. You accept that there are dandelions, but you do not need to let them overgrow. Everything here is up to you. This is your space. No one can take this from you. The same thing can be done with your anxiety. Instead of the dandelions, we're going to grip small, thin blades of grass. You may have done this when you were a child. If you ever sat on the ground with your friends or had a picnic in the park or played sports, you may have ripped the grass out of the soil. You might have torn through the grass and then let go of it, let it float through the air and rejoin the green on the ground like you never even plucked it from the soil.

Blades of grass come out of the ground, some of them longer and some of them shorter. The same can be said about your anxiety. Sometimes, you have bigger things to make you anxious, and sometimes, you have smaller things. Often, it is easy to feel like we are surrounded by our anxiety. Just like your stress and your thoughts, you are in control of it. You have the power to take a deep and calming breath and tell yourself that you are not your anxiety. As you exhale, you let go of that feeling. Take a deep breath in through your nose and tell yourself that you are not your anxiety. You can repeat this in your mind or out loud. It is up to you. I am not my anxiety. Exhale. Release that feeling. Believe in the words you've spoken and let them ring through your body from head to toe. Shake it out. With your eyes closed, shake your head, shaking away those anxieties you carry with you. Shake your shoulders, your hands, and your feet. Imagine that you're covered in water, and you're shaking it all off your body. All of those active feelings and thoughts splash off of your skin, and you let go of them. After you've let go of those anxieties, I want you to open your eyes slowly. Tilt your head backward and look up at the ceiling. I want you to focus on one specific spot. This is another way of practicing the act of letting your thoughts drift away. It's a bit tougher to work on looking at a singular spot, but each time you feel your mind going in a different direction, you simply turn your attention back to that one spot. That's exactly what mindfulness is.

Bringing yourself back to the present moment, to the thing that you're occupied within it, is going to take practice. If you keep at it, you'll be able to do this in the heat of the moment. You'll be able to rewire and train your mind to let go of these thoughts when they're at their worst. Simply shake it off, just as you did a few moments ago. Your heart will pump, bringing you back down to the earth. You'll feel refreshed and free. Breathe in to rebalance yourself, right now and in those moments. Breathe back out. Slowly, take your attention away from the ceiling. Bring yourself back to the present moment. Breathe gently in and out.

When you're ready to, you can return to your day. Shake the meditation out but keep the peace with you. All you need to do is breathe in and out, taking one moment at a time.

Long Guided Meditation 3 (30 Mins)
Relaxation, Stop Thinking, Deep Sleep

THIS IS A LONGER SESSION meant to be listened to when you have more time on your hands to commit to your meditation sessions. You can listen to it over the weekend or while you are on holiday, even if you go away. It will be around half an hour long. By now, I am sure you have grown familiar with the shorter sessions, and you are starting to get used to the longer sessions too. They have either already gotten or are beginning to get easier to sit through. You may have found that you can listen for longer periods of time. These longer sessions may be becoming as natural to sit through as the shorter sessions probably have. Nevertheless, you are more than welcome to keep taking these sessions slowly, one breath and one second at a time. If you only manage half the session or a little more than half the session, that's okay. You can always take on a little more next time. And you can try a little more the time after that. The most important thing for you is to make sure you achieve the goal you set out for. This session is going to help you with relaxation, guide you toward stopping your thinking and helping you to achieve deep sleep. Listen to the sound of my voice as I guide you through this session, while we take you to a place where sleep is easy to come by. I'm going to talk you through it until you're able to let go of the day and drift into the welcoming satisfaction of a restful night, filled with peaceful and harmonious dreams. This is a thirty fifteen-minute session which begins with relaxing the body, aligning the body to your breathing, eventually stopping your thinking, and allowing you to drift off into a deep sleep. To begin with, all the lights should be turned off or dimmed to create a more tranquil environment. Ensure that any other distractions around you have been removed— phone or alarm that might ring, notifications which might ping, and any other such interruptions. Remember, peace and tranquility are keys to relaxation and, eventually, sleep. The fewer distractions you have, the better. You should be lying down. You can lie down on a bed, a sofa, or a meditation mat. The most important part is to make sure that you are comfortable and relaxed, ready to drift off into a deep sleep, where no one will disturb you. Your body should be slack and loose. Start from the positioning of your body while you lie down, making sure that it is at its most comfortable. Slowly, move down each of your limbs, starting at the upper body and cascading down to your legs and feet.

All of your muscles and joints should be drooping as you relax. Let go of all the tension, feeling your body and self relax completely against your place of rest. As always, you are going to start with your breathing. Breathe in deeply through your nose and breathe out gently through your mouth. Let this happen naturally and freely, keeping your breath in for as long as you feel comfortable. As you breathe, release all the tension of the day. Let the stress and excitement ooze from your pores and bones, losing tension in your muscles, draining all the negative energy from your mind and body. You have only good feelings at this moment with each breath. You can feel the comforting sensation of a soft cushion molding around your body, drawing away from the stress and tension like a soothing pillow. You can already feel the energy-sapping away as your body relaxes. Concentrate on and give yourself completely to the current moment. Your day is coming to an end, and it's time to settle in for deep and restful sleep. In the same way that you let your body relax, it is time to let your mind relax. Let go of each bad thought and emotion you have from today. It no longer matters. All that matters right now is this moment. Your body is comfortable in its relaxed state. Your breathing is slow and steady. Now let those feelings and thoughts going through your mind filter away. While you breathe in, your belly pushes inward to capture all the negativity and wakefulness still flowing through your body. Each time you breathe out, you clear those thoughts and feelings out. Feel your chest rise and fall gently with each slow and steady breath. Each continues to clear your body and mind of all unhealthy feelings and thoughts, replacing them with positivity.

If there are any thoughts vying for attention in your mind right now, don't fight their presence. They are supposed to be there. They belong in your mind. Instead of concentrating on them, let them be. Right now, your thoughts are going to be like floating transparent bubbles. You will let each of those thoughts be like a little bubble, similar to the little bubbles in a bottle that kids have; the ones they blow through a wand. The bubbles are light and free, transparent and yet visible, sparkling in the spectrum of rainbow-colored hues. They do not burden but relax. Your thoughts are like these bubbles. Once in the air, they can be popped, or they can float higher and higher into the air until they finally vanish beyond sight. Remember, these thoughts are yours, and you are not getting rid of them, merely letting them slip away from your conscious state. Relaxing your mind as your body is relaxed, drawing in from your thoughts with each breath in, and floating away with each breath out.

Each time a stray thought drifts through the clarity of your mind, let it be nothing more than a bubble floating up and away from you. Do not try and catch or pop the bubbles yourself. You are going to simply let them float away from you. Watch as they go higher and higher until eventually, they disappear into nothingness. Continue your slow and constant breathing while you watch them float away. As each bubble is released, you can feel your mind continue to drift deeper into sleep too. If you inhale deeply enough, you might find that the bubbles move toward you, almost like you're sucking them in. If you exhale, you blow them away from you. This will continue to help clear your mind even more. It also provides a calming and soothing environment for you to rest in. As you feel sleep lull you into its comfortable arms, give your mind a background color. This color is going to be the color of your relaxation. You can choose any- thing you feel comfortable with. The color of lavenders, a light purple, or the color of freshly mown grass, bright green, are both good colors to think about. As you feel your body continues to drift into sleep, this color of relaxation becomes a backdrop for your bubbles, and you can feel your body resting in its presence.

The longer you rest in this serene color, the easier you feel. Your breaths are light and relaxed. Your body is letting go of everything and becoming heavier and heavier against the soft surface beneath your body. Even your thoughts are gentle and quiet, pulling you deeper into sleep. Your eyelids are heavy, and you can't bring yourself to open them. Behind your eye- lids, you can see the color you were thinking of, the color of serenity and sleep. Any thoughts coming to the fore are still bubbles, empty and light as they drift across the background. You can feel yourself drifting off with the thoughts, falling into a deep sleep. The feeling of your own gentle breathing lulls you into a state of quiet clarity. In and out, slow and steady, you breathe deeply and gently. It is like a soothing lullaby, gently guiding you into the embrace of warm and kind sleep. Your arms, legs, hands, feet, and neck all feel heavy as you give yourself over to your dreams. You do not feel any tension in your body, only the softness of your resting place.

If you are still awake, you can turn the device off. When you close your eyes again, you should find that you will be able to easily drift into a deep sleep. Remember to keep breathing in and out deeply through your nose and exhaling gently through your mouth.

CHAPTER 25

HYPNOSIS SESSIONS

Hypnosis 1 (30 Mins)
Relaxation

THIS IS GOING TO BE a thirty-minute guided hypnosis session. The most important thing with this session is to keep an open mind. Go with the flow, listen to my voice, and remember to breathe. It is not always possible to enter a light catatonic state on the first try, but we are going to try and guide you smoothly into this state. Please bear in mind that you are not going to enter any sort of deep catatonic state.

Nothing is going to be altered within the realm of your mind. The whole process is extremely safe, and you are in complete control of it. Hypnosis is nothing but another relaxation method. This session is all about relaxation. I'm going to guide you through the process and help you relax in a much deeper and quicker way than you have ever felt before. For this to work, you need to keep your mind as open as possible and be willing to let go of any resistance. Make yourself comfortable. You should be in a quiet, peaceful space where no one can interrupt you for at least half an hour. You can sit down or lie down, relaxing your shoulders. If you roll your neck, all the tension will seep from your muscles, and you will begin to feel looser as you listen to the sound of my voice. Let my

175

voice bring peace to you, opening your mind. Let go of any inhibitions.

Allow me to guide you and carry you away. We want to use this session to relax you and help you recharge your batteries. This will help you get better at relaxing and letting go. Your back should be straight with hardly any effort or strain put on your muscles and joints. Close your eyes and begin to breathe. You simply need to breathe normally. It may change as the moments' pass. It will happen all on its own. It may grow slower and deeper all on its own. You will find yourself taking a deep breath in through your nose. Afterward, you will exhale gently and let it all out. You simply need to concentrate on your breathing, going with the flow as though it were water in a river, a current ebbing against a bank. If you feel your attention beginning to wander, thoughts drifting into the midst of your mind, simply bring your concentration back to your breathing. Breathe in gently and then out again. Notice the way your stomach pushes out as you fill your lungs with a clear and clean breath. Allow the sensation of relaxation to wash over you, with the same cool water from the flowing river of your thoughts. You may begin to notice small things around you. They'll be things that you normally don't notice, things you look passed. Some of these might even be enjoyable feelings. You might feel the air- brush against your upper lip as you breathe in, cool. It'll feel warmer when you breathe out. Soon, you will be able to follow each breath, and nothing else will mat- ter. Soon, your attention will be focused on nothing but the soothing sensation of your breathing—slow and gentle breaths that spread throughout the muscles and fibers of your body. As the breaths go deeper and deeper, taking you with them, you will begin to hear the gentle sounds of a waterfall. The river of your breath, flowing gently against the bank, is powered by the waterfall. If you feel your attention beginning to wander, bring it back to the waterfall. Notice the way that the whooshing, roaring sound of the water washes away all other thoughts.

All sounds are blocked out as the flow of water splashes down, gently breaking the surface. At this moment, nothing else matters but this time that you are taking for yourself. Your body sinks further and further, as though it is the waterfall. The flow of water is falling deeper into the river below. You switch off all your thoughts and give yourself to the moment. The sound, the cool feeling blowing over your skin, and the deep breaths are all helping you sink into a deeper sense of relaxation. Your body is slowly unwinding, and your mind is following it. You begin to feel more and more relaxed, letting go of all your worries and problems. You don't need to fight any of your negative thoughts right now. They are going to drift away of their own accord, and you are simply going to let go of all of them. I want you to take a few slow, deliberate breaths this time. Fill your lungs with air, letting them expand. And with each exhale, each breath that you let go of, you'll relax more and more. Give your breath a color. This color is the color of your relaxation. Let it fill you up. As it does, notice how the color deepens as it fills you, growing more vibrant the longer you let this breath fill your lungs and expand your belly. Gently set it free, watching the way it grows lighter as it escapes once more. It spreads through your tissues, lighting every tingling part of you up with the colors. You are vibrant and glowing with each breath. The color relaxes you even more. With each breath you release, the color spreads and spreads until it eventually engulfs you. You can see it everywhere. You could even reach out and touch the translucency. You are suspended at this moment, surrounded by the beautiful color of your breath as you continue to breathe deeply in and out. There is no tension. You are floating at this moment, the sensation of complete freedom taking a hold of you. You let yourself go with it. You may even feel an overwhelming sense of happiness wash over you at this moment. Hold onto the color that you've chosen to give to your breath. This color, the color of your relaxation, is how you'll be able to find your way back here. Every time you want to relax, in any time of need, you'll simply breathe deeply in and out and imagine that color. It will be able to transport you to this sense of clarity and serenity. You'll be able to feel it all around you. All you need to do is remember it and give in to the relaxing sensations that come with it. Give yourself to those actions, and it will be easy to do it again and again. You are in total control. Breathe deeply in through your nose and then gently out through your mouth. Your body will grow more comfortable than it's ever been before. You notice the little details about how free your muscles are. You're feeling more relaxed. There's a sensation that flows through your body, making your limbs feel heavy. From the top of your head, tingling through every inch of your body all the way down to the very tips of your toes, you'll feel no more tension. You release the tension from your jaw. Your body feels as though it is loaded with the lead with every word I speak. This is the weight of peace and serenity filling you from the inside out. You are glowing with a feeling of great contentment and calmness. The feeling of relaxation flowing through your body is almost like a gentle massage as it moves through your muscles, led entirely by your own mind, making its way down your spine as it goes. It is nearly time to come back, but remember that you can do this on your own. The next time you relax, you choose to relax like this. You can relax far more quickly than before. You will relax easier than before. Your relaxation will be much deeper. Each time you choose to relax like this, it will come more naturally, and you will find yourself slipping into this place with no effort. When you return to the present moment, you are going to slowly start to notice the surroundings. You are going to be able to feel the cushion beneath you, the soft- ness and comfort your body sinks into and relaxes against. You are going to bring back all the pleasant sensations you felt in this sensation, whether it is the light feeling in your chest or the way your breath stretched your diaphragm. You are slowly returning to wakefulness. Your energy levels are rising, and you are feeling more invigorated than before. You are more aware and alert than when we started the session. The feeling begins to return to your muscles. They slowly come back to life. You can stretch your limbs out, loosening your joints. Slowly, you open your eyes. At the first light in the room, you are feeling more alert than ever.

You feel as though you have just woken from a deep and refreshing sleep, and you are ready to face your day once more.

Hypnosis 2 (30 Mins)
Stop Overthinking, Anxiety, and Stress

THIS IS GOING TO BE a thirty-minute guided hypnosis session. The most important thing with this session is to keep an open mind. Go with the flow, listen to my voice, and remember to breathe. It is not always possible to enter a light catatonic state on the first try, but we are going to try and guide you smoothly into this state. Please bear in mind that you are not going to enter any sort of deep catatonic state. Nothing is going to be altered within the realm of your mind. The whole process is extremely safe, and you are in control of it. I want you to get comfortable. You should be sitting or lying down. Sit back and let your shoulders go slack, relaxing against the cushion behind you. Gently close your eyes and release all the tension from your muscles. All the muscles in your body begin to feel looser and looser. Listen to the sound of my voice. Let it soothe you. Release all your inhibitions and open your mind. Allow yourself, in body and mind, to be carried away. Allow yourself to be lulled into a sense of calming security. Sway your head back and forth by the smallest amount, just enough for you to feel the heaviness of your skull. Move it back and forth, slower and slower until you feel that you're starting to get more relaxed. You can stop when you've reached that point. Rest your head back. Take a deep breath in and then let it out. Breathe in

Hypnosis Sessions

deeply through your nose. Now breathe out through your mouth. Continue to breathe deeply as you slowly move your focus to your toes. Curl your toes as you feel the warm sensation of relaxation move from the very tips of your toes upward, toward your ankles, and finally, up to your calves. All the tension in your muscles disappears as the sensation moves upward. It moves past your thighs and toward the curves of your knees. It continues to travel higher and higher. Notice that your legs are feeling heavy, and you are feeling calmer than before. Give in to the sensation coursing through your body from the toes upward.

Drift into a deeper feeling of serenity and tranquility with every breath that you take. Breathe in. Now breathe out. Slowly, deeply. Breathe in. Breathe out. That peaceful sensation of relaxation continues to make it's way higher, past your waist and your stomach. It works its way over your ribs, heading toward your chest. The feeling calms you and soothes you. All your worries begin to fade away, and you let them go, the same way you let go of your shoulders and back as the muscles in them loosen even more. Your arms are beginning to relax too, your elbows and your wrists, your hands and your fingers. Let them. Let go of the desire to fight the relaxing sensation. Release the control over your body and give in to the calming sensation. Relax your neck, your jaw, your face, and your forehead. Realize how good it feels to let go of all that tension. At this moment, nothing else matters. There is nowhere for you to be. You only need to be here, at this moment, letting the relaxing sensation wash over your body. Your thoughts drift away, but you let them. You don't try to follow or catch them. They simply float through and pass on their way out. With each breath you take, you are feeling more and more serene. Breathe in, invit- ing peace and harmony to your soul. Breathe out, exhaling all the negative energy and control. Take note of how good it feels to be so relaxed. I'm going to count now. Let my voice lull you. You are safe and relaxed. Ten...your body is entirely relaxed. Nine...you are in a peaceful, calm environment. Eight...you can feel the warmth and love of those who care about you, engulfing your senses. Seven...each sound that you hear around you puts you into an even deeper state of relaxation.

Six...you inhale all of the good in the world with each breath you take. Five...you exhale all the bad, blowing away all of your stress and anxiety with each breath out. Four...you feel your body slipping even deeper. Three...relax and allow your mind to become even heavier. Two...keep calm, slipping ever deeper into the feeling of relaxation. One...you feel yourself slipping all the way down, as deep as you can go. You are safe and relaxed. Let yourself feel safe and relaxed in this space. Your imagination leads you to a beautiful place where you can escape to relax. This is a soft, gentle place that you wander through. It looks like the woods, dense on either side with rays of sunlight shining through the canopy of branches high above your head. The leaves of the trees rustle in the gentle breeze. In your mind's eye, you can visualize this tranquil place. Feel the soft, spongy grass underfoot. You're floating toward this place, moving closer and closer until you finally start to notice the details of your surroundings. You can see the colors of the grass and of the bark and of the leaves on the branches of trees. You can see the tall shapes of the trees, sentries that guard over and protect you. When you finally arrive, you can hear sounds all around you. Leaves are rustling gently as the breeze blows against them. Birds are gently chirping somewhere in the distance, singing a happy song. This place is peaceful. You can feel it dance over every nerve ending in your body, making every part of you tingle. The feeling of its kind and caressing touch on your skin makes you feel completely at peace. In this place, there is no such thing as time. This is where you come to the center and balance yourself. Here, you won't have to worry about anything at all. As you walk along the forest path, I want you to take a deep breath. You're going to notice something. It looks like a carving in the wood of one of the beautiful trees. You make your way toward it. Breathe out at the sight of it. There is a word carved neatly into the bark, just one single word.

The word is the name of this place. Just the sound of it brings you here. It's a soothing, serene word. Look closely at the carving in the bark and identify the word. It's a word of your choosing. This word comes to you and you alone. I want you to remember this word because every time you are feeling even the smallest amount of anxiety or stress, you're going to call on this word. Every time that you say the word out loud or in your mind, you're going to be reminded of this place. The amazing feeling of relaxation that you feel washing over every inch of you will come back to you. Hold onto the word so that you can always use it when you need to. Take a deep breath in through your nose. Look around at the forest surrounding you, the bark of the trees and the green of the leaves. Take in the deep blue sky, free of clouds, and the soft feel of the undergrowth beneath your feet. Notice how relaxed this place makes you feel. Notice how relaxed you are at this very moment. Notice how calming the sensations in your body are.

I am going to count to five. When I reach five, you are going to be fully alert. You will feel refreshed and rejuvenated in every possible way, mind and body. One...you are feeling incredible. The sensations running through you are good. Two...you feel free and fresh, as though your visit to your special place refreshed you the same way a shower would have. Three...you start to notice the sounds and temperature of the room around you. Four...the feeling in your fingers and your toes are beginning to return, making you more aware of your body than before. Five...you are now awake and alert. Take a deep breath in. Exhale. Stretch your limbs out. Say your word. Say the word that was on the bark in the forest out loud. If your mind wandered or you fell asleep during the session, that is all right. It's perfectly normal. Each time you practice these sessions, you'll be making them a little easier, and you'll be able to last a little longer than before. You can use this technique to relax at any time that you want to.

Whenever you find yourself in an anxious or stressful situation, all you need to do is repeat your word out loud to yourself. You'll find that an enormous clarity washes over your mind and your body will be able to easily relax.

Hypnosis 3 (30 Mins)

Relaxation, Stop Thinking, Deep Sleep

THIS IS A THIRTY-MINUTE guided hypnosis session. The most important thing to remember as you listen during this session is to keep an open mind. Go along with the flow, listen to my voice, and most importantly, remember to breathe. Do not be discouraged if you do not enter a light catatonic state on the first try. We will be slowly working toward smoothly transitioning you into this state as we go along. Do bear in mind that you will not enter into any sort of deep hypnotic state during this session. Nothing within the realm of your mind will be altered or negatively affected. The entire process is safe, and you will maintain control throughout. The goal is to help your mind flit into a state of fatigue when you need to, helping you sleep easier and better with less effort.

To begin, let us start with a simple breathing and visualization exercise. Make sure that you are in a comfortable position, lying down on a meditation mat, sofa, or bed, as long as your body is in a relaxed position and prepared for sleep. Remove all distractions around you which might pull your attention away from listening. Once you are set, close your eyes and listen only to my voice. We will now begin the breathing exercise.

Take a deep breath slowly through your nose, holding it in for five seconds.

Five.

Four.

Three.

Two.

One.

And exhale slowly out through your mind, feeling the air rush out of your longs. Keep your breathing relaxed and do not strain your lungs. Keep your breathing natural and normal as once again you draw your breath in through your nose. Keep it in and exhale. As you steady your breathing, shut your eyes to the world until you are lost in the darkness behind your eyelids. This is the first state of relaxation. Imagine each breath flowing from your nose, flowing like a waterfall through your body, filling it right down, circulating around your system, and escaping once again through your mouth. Imagine now that this waterfall flows into a quiet river. Follow the river in your mind. The water does not rush by and does not make a noise. It flows slow, steady, and continuously along, and as it moves, you can feel the rest of your body relax into it. All tension in your body slackens and loosens, relaxing every muscle in your body from top to bottom. It seeps into your muscles, relaxing every nerve and fiber. Each time you breathe, you feel the tension inside your body melt away as the river in your mind flows and guides you into a state of complete relaxation. We will continue this for five more seconds. With each count, you feel all the knots loosen from your mind and body, all tensions and stresses evaporating, guiding you to relax further and further. I will begin the count. Five...your hands and fingers are relaxed and open. Four...your body begins to grow more comfortable. Your eyelids grow heavier. Three...your breathing grows steadier and calmer. Two...you You begin to feel your body sink deeper into a relaxed state. One...all the stress and tension have drained out of your body, making you feel relaxed and ready for sleep. Follow your quiet and peaceful river toward a wide lake—a calm, smooth lake. This lake is your mind and body at its most relaxed state, as calm as your continued breathing. Let your mind drift along the calm waters, your consciousness falling deeper and deeper into a peaceful state. Your lake is only as calm as your thoughts. Although it is serene and peaceful, there are thoughts that still cross your mind. They appear like ripples on the surface of the water, disturbing it. Do not let the ripples worry you. These are your day's thoughts and stresses attempting to sink back into your lake of tranquility. With each ripple swirling into existence, imagine that they ripple in time with your breathing. When you breathe in, imagine that you are drawn in-breath is a first swirl of thought unsettling the waters, and as you breathe out, you watch the ripple float further and further away from the lake, returning it to its serene state. Let us count down from twenty, and with each count, you let another ripple of thought float away to the edges, smoothing your thoughts as they smooth the waters. And with each dispersed ripple, your mind feels more and more at peace with itself, each time pulling you deeper into a calm state of sleep, your eyelids feeling heavier with each one. Twenty...your most pressing thought is only a small ripple. Nineteen...it is carried away. You can already feel lighter. Eighteen...your next pressing thought is only a small ripple. Seventeen...it is carried away. Your mental burdens are already easing. Sixteen...as each ripple disappears, you feel more rested and content with life.

Fifteen...sleep pulls you closer. Your body is feeling its most relaxed, your mind composed and happy. Continue on dispersing thoughts as ripples. You are already feeling refreshed. You can already feel your body relax comfortably around you. There are peace and tranquility. You float on your lake peacefully. Lying in your space of rest and comfort, floating easily atop your quiet, calm lake, you can still hear my voice. It continues to soothe and guide your consciousness but never disrupting it. You are at greater peace. Any thought that drifts into your thoughts now barely affects your rest. My voice is merely a guide. You can feel your eyelids too heavy to lift. Your body is in total relaxation. It floats over the lake and looks forward to waking. In these last few minutes, we will prepare your mind for wakefulness. Above your lake is a beautiful night sky, bright and clear. Your mind knows that after this beautiful night is over, your body will feel refreshed and ready for a new day. You will be carried back from the lake along your tranquil river and into fulness. But for now, you are a boat that awaits the shore. You can see the shore in the distance, and you wait for it patiently. I will count now from fifteen downward. With each count, your body and mind will begin to prepare to store all the energy and positivity it requires for another day—a productive and fruitful day with an energized body and willing mind. Your consciousness has not completely slipped into sleep yet, but you're right on at its edge and falling deeper and deeper still. I will begin the count. Fifteen...you sift through your mind and body for any remaining tension. Fourteen...your continued and steadied breathing once again flows from river to lake. Thirteen...anything that prevents sleep is simply washed away. Your body is at peace. Twelve...any ripples of thought that appear are easily and quickly dispersed. Your mind is at peace. Eleven...the lake around lulls you to sleep like a quiet melodious lullaby.

Ten...with each continued breath, your body revitalizes itself, drawing in its inner strength and storing it within you. Nine...your mind easily aligns your thoughts and actions into understandable and easily distinguishable thoughts. Eight...together, your mind and bodywork toward correcting any negativity and re- placing it with all the positive energy surrounding you. Seven...the energy circulates your sleeping body, wrapping around you like a warm and comfortable cocoon waiting to be released upon waking. Six...your eyelids have already truly begun to shut, and sleep beckons you. Five...you are relaxed. Four...you are at peace.

Three...you are ready for a new day. Two...when you awake the next day, you will be fully refreshed both in body and mind. One...sleep is now ready to accept you.

If you are still awake, you can turn off the device and close your eyes again. Sleep will welcome you easily and prepare you for a full day of positive productivity. You will be able to face it feeling completely refreshed and revitalized.

CHAPTER 26

DAILY AFFIRMATIONS

25 Daily Affirmations to Cope with Stress and Anxiety (10 Mins)

IT CAN SEEM IMPOSSIBLE to get over your anxiety, especially when you get anxious about getting over it. It's very easy to obsess about this and very difficult to resist the urge to scream at your own mind. Unfortunately, we know that this doesn't work. You might even find that it makes you feel worse. Not to worry. There are kinder ways to talk to yourself, and these can help you soothe your mind. I'm going to take you through twenty-five positive affirmations to help you cope with your stress and anxiety. In times of need, you can repeat these affirmations to yourself, or you can run through them in your mind. These are going to be especially helpful when combined with your meditation and hypnosis sessions.

Relax. Close your eyes. Listen to my voice.

Repeat after Me

1. I know that I am not my anxiety or stress.

2. My stress and anxiety are temporary.

3. I am strong, and I can make it through this.

4. I cannot control everything, and it is not my responsibility to do so.

5. I am taking one step at a time on the road of personal growth.

6. I do not need to let these feelings and thoughts bring me down.

7. I accept that the only constant in my life—and anyone's—is changing.

8. The challenges that come my way bring opportunities with them.

9. I am learning to let go of my worries.

10. I take a time-out of each day to relieve my stress, and this is important.

11. I am working on making my life more balanced and enjoyable.

12. I choose to release the bad of the past and look forward to the good that will come my way.

13. I am learning that it is okay that I have the strength to heal and grow.

14. I accept that everything happens for a reason, and things are working out

15. the way they are meant to right now.

16. No matter what, I am doing the best that I can do.

17. There is no such thing as a mistake, only a lesson to learn from.

18. I inhale all the good with each breath I take, and I exhale all the bad.

19. My mind is becoming a tranquil thing as I learn to clear it.

20. I have survived this before, and I will survive it again.

21. I am worthy of love, and so is everyone else.

22. As each new day passes, I am slowly becoming the best version of myself there is.

23. I do not need anyone else's approval. I know that my mind and body are doing all they can for me.

24. There is nothing that I can't overcome.

25. I need to keep in mind that I have the power to say no and to walk away from things that are not good for my mental and physical health.

26. Setting aside this time is good for my well-being.

25 Daily Affirmations to Stop Thinking and Become Mindful (10 Mins)

OVERTHINKING CAN WREAK havoc on your mind by overwhelming you and making you feel like you have no control. It isn't easy to rid yourself of something that is always in your own mind. You needn't feel like there is no way to stop these thoughts from ruling your head and your days. Practicing mindfulness is an excellent way to overcome obsessive thoughts. You need to focus your attention on the here and now, ensuring that you are completely aware of each moment in your life. All the positive feelings that we want to feel can only be discovered in the present moment. One of the most important things is to realize that these are your thoughts. You are the only one who has power over them, but this will also take commitment and dedication. These affirmations are going to help you stop thinking and be more mindful.

I want you to close your eyes and relax. Stay positive while you listen to my voice. Think of happiness, inspiration, love, and the good things that are going to come your way.

Repeat after Me

1. I have full control over my own thoughts.

2. It is up to me to relax under the strain of mental pressure, and I can do this.

3. I am going to cut the cords of my obsessive thoughts and let them go.

4. I can stop allowing my obsessive thoughts to classify me as less than I am.

5. It is within my power to take a step back and assess my thoughts.

6. By focusing on the present, I am able to bring myself a sense of calm and clarity.

7. I can concentrate on the now and keep my thoughts from drifting to negative places.

8. I let go of all the negativity of the past and bring myself forward to the current moment in time.

9. I breathe in and out and take each day one moment at a time without fear orworry about the past and future.

10. I am making an effort not to judge others who are quietly battling with their own journey of self-improvement.

11. Life is too short to worry about small things.

12. I only have one life, so I shouldn't overthink and waste the little time I have when I could be enjoying it instead.

13. I will make decisions from a healthy space.

14. I put all my effort and attention into whatever I am doing.

15. I have the freedom to make my own choices and decisions.

16. With each day that passes, I become more liberated.

17. I will look for solutions rather than problems.

18. I will make an effort to keep an open mind.

19. The best way to appreciate this life is to live in the present moment.

20. I am much bigger and much better than the mere scale of my thoughts.

21. The only thing that really matters is this moment right now.

22. I make each second count.

23. Time is on my side.

24. Right now is the best time of my life.

25. I practice mindfulness and meditation each day.

25 Daily Affirmations to Relax and Improve Sleep (10 Mins)

PEACE CAN BE DIFFICULT to obtain. There are so many disruptions in our days and our heads that they can simmer to boiling point. These feelings may not leave you even when all you seek is a quiet night's rest. These affirmations can help put you into a frame of mind that is peaceful and relaxed, instead of tense and edgy. If you apply them consistently, they will help you fall asleep and have a well-rested night far easier. Healthy sleeping routines and patterns can help you lead a healthier and more balanced life.

I want you to close your eyes and listen to the sound of my voice. Let go of all the stress of the day with a few deep breaths in and out. You deserve to wake up feel- ing nice and refreshed in the morning.

Repeat after Me in Your Mind to Create a More Peaceful Environment

1. I release all that happened today.

2. I am in complete control of my sleeping habits and patterns.

3. Relaxing before sleep will ensure that I sleep deeply.

4. I am slowly transforming into a deep sleeper.

5. I welcome dreams full of harmony, coolness, and serenity.

6. I keep only positive feelings and emotions of the day.

7. I am clearing my mind with each breath, letting the day slip away.

8. I am light enough to let the tranquility of sleep carry me and take me fromthis place.

9. All my muscles are becoming looser as I release the tension of the day.

10. With each breath, I invite harmony and serenity into my life and my rest.

11. I am going to wake up feeling rejuvenated and refreshed.

12. I am going to have a deep and restful night.

13. Everything that I did today was more than enough.

14. I welcome the embrace of deep sleep.

15. My mind is light and peaceful, free of all negative energy.

16. I am willing to forgive anything and everything in the past.

17. I am calm in the knowledge that I do the best that I can each day.

18. My body and my mind are nourished by the serenity of sleep.

19. Each part of me is growing heavier and heavier with the prospect of a good

20. night's rest.

21. I am comfortable and relaxed in the sanctuary of my soft bed.

22. My chest gently rises and falls with each breath, like the soft tides of the sea

23. flowing and ebbing on the shore of a beach.

24. I allow the natural process of sleep to caress my mind with kind and tender hands.

25. My mind is still, like the surface of a lake beneath the moonlight.

26. I am surrounded by the warm energy of the people I love.

27. Each time I exhale, I let go of the stress and anxiety of the day, allowing myself to fall into a deep and relaxing sleep.

FAQ'S

1. Is gastric sleeve surgery a cure for obesity?

   Bear in mind that this procedure is not the ultimate cure for obesity, by any means. Gastric sleeve surgery is merely a jump-start or tool for the patient to address chronic weight issues and start on a healthy lifestyle that involves a solid diet plan and ample exercise.

2. How much weight can I expect to lose? You need to know how much weight you should expect to lose after the surgery, then there are some simple calculations. You will lose somewhere around 60% of the extra weight over two years, with the majority of it likely coming off in the first year.

   Long-term weight loss, however, is more dependent on what you eat, how much you exercise, etc. rather than which procedure(s) you undertake. It is possible to gain all the weight back.

3. So, will I gain back the weight lost after surgery?

   The possibility cannot be ruled out. The whole point of the gastric sleeve surgery is that you lose weight after the removal of a portion of your stomach, thereby decreasing the sheer capacity of your stomach to hold and digest food. However, this procedure should be complemented by healthy dietary and exercise habits for you to remain trim. If the patient won't change their lifestyle after the surgery, then the lost weight is regained by the body in due course.

4. Will my stomach stretch after surgery? It can stretch, but it depends on how much you normally feed it. For an occasional large meal, your stomach can stretch to accommodate it and then get back to its smaller size. However, if you continue to give it large meals (or meals too large for the size your stomach will be), then it can and will stretch without returning to its smaller size. If you stretch it back out, you eat more food. When you eat more food, you gain weight.

CONCLUSION

While telling a person to adopt the mentally healthy traits is an excellent way to develop mental toughness, it may not always be enough. In a way, it's a bit like telling a person to be healthy; you need to eat correctly, exercise, and get plenty of rest. Such advice is good and even correct. However, it lacks an individual specificity that can leave a person feeling unsure of exactly what to do. Fortunately, several practices can create a clear plan of how to achieve mental toughness. These practices are like the actual recipes and exercises needed to eat right and get plenty of activities. By adopting these practices in your daily work, you will begin to find yourself trapped in mental resilience in every job you do and in every cnvironment. Keep your emotions in check

The most important thing you can do in developing mental toughness is to keep your emotions in check. People who fail to take control of their feelings allow their feelings to control them. More often than not, this takes the form of people driven by rage, fear, or both. Whenever people allow their emotions to manage them, they let their emotions control their decisions, words, and actions. However, when you keep your emotions in check, you take control of your choices, comments, and activities, thereby taking control of your life overall.

To keep your emotions in check, you have to learn to subside your feelings be- fore reacting to a situation. Therefore, instead of speaking when you are angry, or deciding when you are frustrated, take a few minutes to allow your emotions to settle down. Take a moment to simply sit down, breathe deeply, and let your energies to restore balance. Only when you feel calm and in control should you make your decision, speak your mind, or take any action. Practice detachment

Another critical element for mental toughness is what is known as detachment. It is when you remove yourself emotionally from the particular situation that is going on around you. Even if the condition affects you directly, remaining detached is a very positive thing. The most significant benefit of detachment is that it pre- vents an emotional response to the situation at hand. It is incredibly helpful when things are not going according to plan.

Practicing detachment requires a great deal of effort at first. After all, most people are programmed to feel emotionally attached to the events going on around them at any given time. One of the best ways to practice detachment is to tell your- self that the situation isn't permanent. What causes a person to feel fear and frustration when faced with a negative situation is that they think the problem is permanent. When you realize that even the worst events are temporary, you avoid creating a negative emotional response. Another way to become detached is to determine why you feel attached to the situation in the first place. If someone is saying or doing something to hurt your feelings, understand that their words and actions reflect them, not you. As long as you don't feed into their negativity, you won't experience the pain they are trying to cause. It is valid for anything you share. By not providing a negative situation or event with negative emotions, you prevent that situation from connecting to you. It allows you to exist within an adverse event without being affected by it.

Accept what is beyond your control acceptance is one of the cornerstones of mental toughness. It can take the form of accepting yourself for who you are and accepting others for who they are, but it can also take the way of getting what is beyond your control. When you learn to buy things that cannot be changed, you will rewrite your thoughts on how you react to every situation you encounter. The fact is that most of the stress and anxiety that ordinary people feel causes by the inability to change certain things. Once you learn to accept those things you can't change, you permanently eliminate all of that harmful stress and anxiety.

While accepting what is beyond your control will take a little practice, it is relatively easy. The trick is to simply ask yourself if you can do anything to change the situation at hand. If the answer is 'no,' simply let it go. Rather than wasting time and energy fretting about what you can't control, adopt the mantra, "It is what it is." It might seem careless at first, but you will realize that it is a real sign of mental strength after a while. By accepting what is beyond your control, you conserve your energy, thoughts, and time for those things you can affect, thereby making your efforts more effective and worthwhile.   Always be prepared another way to build mental toughness is always to prepare. If you allow life to take you from one event to another, you will feel lost, uncertain, and unprepared for the experiences you encounter. When you take the time to prepare for what is about to happen, you will always maintain a sense of control over the situation. There are two ways to be ready, and they are equally crucial for developing mental toughness.   The first way to be prepared is to prepare your mind at the beginning of every day. It takes the form of you taking time in the morning to focus your mind on who you are, what you are capable of, and your outlook on life in general. Whether you refer to this time as mediation, contemplation, or daily affirmations, the basic principle is the same. You only need to focus on your beliefs and the qualities you pursue. It will keep you grounded in your ideals throughout the day, helping you make the right choices regardless of what life throws your way.   The second way to always be prepared is to take the time to prepare yourself for the situation at hand. If you must give a presentation, make sure to give yourself enough time to prepare. Read carefully the information you want to provide, choose the materials you want to use, and even take a moment to make sure you have the exact clothes you want to wear. When you go into a situation fully pre-pared, you increase your self-confidence, giving you an added edge. Additionally, you will eliminate the stress and anxiety that results from feeling unprepared.

Take the time to embrace success one of the problems many negatively minded people experience is that they never take the time to appreciate success when it comes to their way. Sometimes they are too afraid of jinxing that success actually to recognize it.

However, most of the time, they cannot embrace success because their mindset is simply too negative for such positive action. By contrast, mentally healthy people always take the time to embrace the sensations that come their way. It serves to build their sense of confidence and their feeling of satisfaction with how things are going. You experience the success of any kind, make sure you take a moment to recognize it. You can create an external statement, such as going out for drinks, treating yourself to a nice lunch, or some similar expression of gratitude.

Alternatively, you can simply take a quiet moment to reflect on the success and all the effort that went into making it happen. There is no right or wrong way to embrace success. You just need to find a method that works for you. The trick to welcoming success is in not letting it go to your head. Rather than praising your efforts or actions, appreciate the fact that things went well. Also, be sure to enjoy those whose help contributed to your success. Be happy with what you have Contentment is another element that is critical for mental toughness. To develop happiness, you have to learn how to be happy with what you have. It doesn't mean that you eliminate ambition or the desire to achieve tremendous success. In- stead, you show gratitude for the positives that currently exist. After all, the only way you will appreciate the fulfillment of your dreams truly is if you can first under- stand your life the way it is.

One example of this is learning to appreciate your job. It is true whether you like work or not. Even if you hate your job and want to find another job, take some time to appreciate the fact that you have your first job. The truth is that you could be jobless, which would create all sorts of problems in your life. So, even if you hate your job, learn to appreciate it for what it is. It goes for everything in your life. Be happy with who you are   In addition to appreciating what you have, you should always be happy with who you are. Again, this doesn't mean that you should settle for who you are and not try to improve your life; instead, it means that you should learn to appreciate who you are at every moment. There will always be issues that you want to fix in your life, and things you know you could do better. If you focus on the wrong things, you will always see yourself in a negative light. However, when you learn to appreciate the right parts of your personality, you can pursue self-improvement with a sense of pride, hope, and optimism for who you will become as you begin to fulfill your true potential.

www.ingramcontent.com/pod-product-compliance
Lightning Source LLC
Chambersburg PA
CBHW060319030426
42336CB00011B/1127